CAUGHT-IN-THE-MIDDLE MANAGEMENT

TAKING CARE OF YOURSELF — AND YOUR ORGANIZATION

Written by:
Clyde W. Jackson
Robert L. Slaton, Ed.D., FACMPE
Bob Manning

Illustrations by:
Lyle Slaton

Published by:
Medical Group Management Association
104 Inverness Terrace East
Englewood, CO 80112
(303) 799-1111

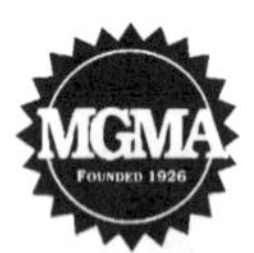

Medical Group Management Association
104 Inverness Terrace East
Englewood, CO 80112

ISBN # 1-56829-075-6

Pam,
you're a very special
person & a dear
friend. I miss you
& hope you move
to Louisville soon.
Love
Robert

TABLE of CONTENTS

Table of contents

ACKNOWLEDGEMENTS

Among countless people owed debts of gratitude, the authors particularly acknowledge those who appear in this book as composite characters such as Dr. Godley, Jonathan, Lauree, Mr. Sam, Ms. Sharp, Ms. Short, and Tim. The authors dedicate this book to them and to the many family members, friends, and colleagues who (despite our strong resistance) actually did manage to teach us a thing or two.

The book would not have been possible without the support of the Medical Group Management Association staff: **Fred E. Graham, II, Ph.D., FACMPE/CAE, Senior Vice President/Chief Operating Officer, Barbara U. Hamilton, M.A., Library Resource Center Director**; and the assistance of **Alys and Brian Novak, Discovery Communications, Inc.**

INTRODUCTION

Preparing for battle

Hammered. Stretched. Squeezed. Pressured, pulled, tugged, trapped. That's how many managers in health care organizations might describe themselves today. Like the rope in a tug of war, managers live in the battle zone between strong, opposing forces. Many managers feel themselves unraveling, stretched to the point of breaking, caught in the middle between an unsatisfying present and an uncertain future. Their predicament:

- Managers must work every day as though the wolf of unemployment was at their door. But these days everyone knows their job can be eliminated without notice through downsizing, merger, or acquisition — no matter how good a job they have been doing. The wolf is on the inside, not the outside.

- In an effort to control the bottom line, managers must cut expenses. Yet they know that short-term cuts can hamstring the organization in the long term. Who will be blamed? Take an obvious guess: the managers.

- To cut costs and increase revenues, managers must ask their employees to work harder and to do more — often for no increase in pay. Managers must maintain the commitment and enthusiasm of a core group of key employees, while laying off those employees' friends and co-workers.

- Managers must make commitments on the basis of signals from senior management, then sometimes renege on the commitments when conditions change. Managers must support the "party line," even when they suspect that elements of the party line are incomplete, inappropriate, wrong, or untrue.

Most of this is not new. Managers have always faced challenges — that's what keeps them employed. But what *is* new for health care managers nowadays is the variety and intensity of these challenges. The landscape of health care has become a fertile breeding ground where new forms of business competition spring hungrily to life almost every day. Like predatory viruses, they mutate in response to constantly changing regulatory and market environments. They invade. They maraud. They feed on their hosts.

C. Everett Koop, the former Surgeon General, has said that health care in the 1990's will be shaped by forces similar to those that shaped airlines and banking in the 1980's. Rapid growth of national providers and managed care plans, emerging technologies, changes in the rules for government funding, aggressive health care marketing, outcomes analysis, and many other factors are at play, and will cause enormous upheaval in the industry. There will be bloodletting as these forces vie for the privilege of sucking money out of the established health care system. There will be disruptions to the careers of good people.

In this book, we will help you manage in that environment.

How? By preparing you for battle. By painting a realistic picture of the opportunities and the dangers in today's world. By helping you recognize who has the most control and influence over your job, your job performance, and your future: you!

CHAPTER 1

Caught-in-the-middle management

A wise old story ends with the moral, "Be careful what you wish for, because it may come true." Many health care managers wish they could escape the anxiety of their jobs. Unfortunately these days, some people get that wish — when they lose their jobs.

As the introduction mentions, managers are always caught in the middle. We should all be so lucky. "In the middle" is where the action is — and where good employment opportunities can be found. So this book does not try to tell managers how to escape from the "middle." Quite the contrary. As long as you are in the middle, no matter how bad things are, at least you have a job.

Is that the best you can expect? We hope not. This book takes the optimistic position that life in the middle can (often) be sane, orderly, secure, and rewarding for managers.

This book claims that people can achieve those things through good *management*. In other words, the authors believe all managers are caught in the middle, but some people find ways to *manage* their situations better than others. Those people prosper as a result. But we don't just mean those people do a good job managing their offices or clinics or departments; we also mean they do a good job managing their *careers*.

Some readers may smile when they realize that the title of this book has nothing to do with "middle management." The book is not about middle management. Certainly it is about management, but the title refers to management techniques that can be useful for all people who are caught in the middle, usually between conflicting obligations. You don't have to be in "middle management" to be caught in the middle.

So in this book we will use the phrase "caught-in-the-middle management" to describe techniques, theories, perspectives — perhaps what might be called an outlook, or an approach, or a management path — that can lead to success by improving the way you manage yourself, your job, and your career.

Three make-or-break factors

The health care delivery system in America today is stressed. Does that mean that there is stress in your little corner of this massive system? Almost certainly. The late

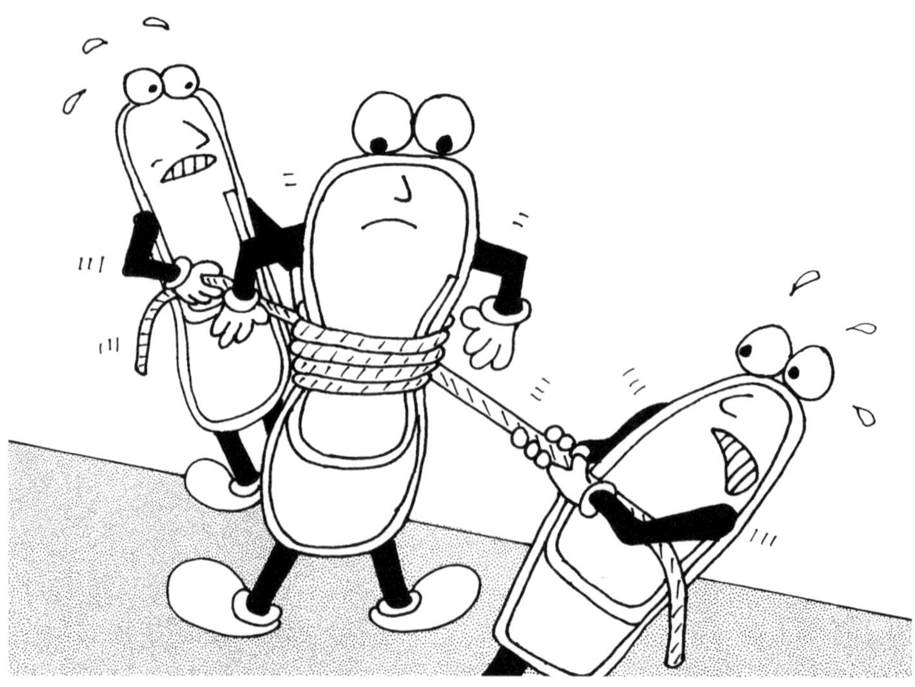

Tip O'Neill used to say that all politics is local politics. Similarly, all stress is local stress. What's happening in the industry will affect your organization, your employees, your job. If you have already come to that realization, congratulations. You have passed step one of caught-in-the-middle managing.

Caught-in-the-middle managing focuses on three fundamental activities for managers:

- View the next 18 months as the most critical period in your organization's history — and as the most important period of your career;

- Get the facts. In other words, relentlessly gather and analyze information about your business and your career. Then develop worst-case scenarios for your organization — and for your career; and

- Take care of yourself, so you can take care of your organization.

We will introduce these ideas in this chapter, and will deal with them in greater detail in individual chapters later in the book.

The crunch period

First, caught-in-the-middle managing views the next 1 to 18 months as the most critical period you will know. Treat that period as though it makes or breaks your organization and your career. It is that middle period, between the way things are and the way they will be. If you have any chance at all to affect the future, you will affect it during that middle period.

By way of clarification, when we say "the next 18 months," what we mean is a rolling 18 months. In other words, the period begins anew every month. It does not end a year and a half from now, at which time a new period begins.

Eighteen months from now, 18 months from every "now," is the critical middle period when you make or break your career and when your organization thrives or fails. A large managed care provider can set your organization on a downward spiral in the next 1 to 18 months. You can learn a new set of skills to compete in managed care in that period. You can read the tea leaves and see how to strengthen your organization in that amount of time, or you can read the tea leaves and see that your organization cannot afford you if something doesn't change. You can find a new job in a year and a half.

Go for the facts

The second principle of caught-in-the-middle management is summed up by the phrase "Get the facts, or the facts will get you." Managers need to be insatiably curious. They must develop an appetite for facts. Objectivity is the order of the day, and e-v-e-r-y-t-h-i-n-g about the business must be available for examination. In addition, self-appraisal is required, even if it is painful. And worst-case scenarios must be routinely reviewed, not just for business projects, but for personal and career projects as well.

Why this emphasis on fact-finding? The primary reason is the simple, undeniable truth that the business world runs on the fuel of information. The more, and the more accurate, the better. The fundamental business activities of planning, organizing, directing, evaluating, monitoring...were long ago proven to work better in an environment rich in factual information.

But there is another, more subtle reason for an emphasis on getting the facts. It has to do with how human beings live and work and relate to each other. It has to do with credibility.

Just as business activities flourish in an environment rich in factual information, so do employees respond to honesty and openness. This human need is particularly evident during periods of rapid change. Whenever you hear talk about organizational "reshaping," the focus is usually on the changes needed within a business or industry to ensure its survival. In other words, the focus is on the organization, not on individuals. The human needs of those affected by the changes can go largely unmet, during and after the changes...often leaving senior managers to wonder why subordinates feel so little loyalty to them and to the organization.

Caught-in-the-middle management acknowledges that by necessity there will always be layoffs, downsizing, and other unpleasant or painful aspects of business life. But open discussion of the human toll is a vital step toward reducing the pressure and pain. That means managers must uncover and understand and discuss openly the "soft facts." They must deal with the truths about the human beings within their organizations — just as thoroughly as managers must dig for the hard facts about cash flow, productivity, and competition.

Another benefit: When managers are familiar with the facts, they are less likely to be surprised or shocked by sudden events, and they are more objective and effective. Managers must become steeled to the unpleasant truths of the workplace. A co-worker is a power-hungry back-stabber? Well, better to know that early so you can protect yourself and your people. The company has been borrowing heavily, and profits are still lagging? Well, let's calculate how long before the axe will fall, so we can make some plans...

You see the point.

This type of constant questioning makes the important task of doing worst-case scenarios easy. When you accurately describe the worst case and then manage for it, all your surprises are pleasant. Planning for the worst case builds in a safety net. Planning for the best case leaves no safety net and ensures that your surprises will be nasty.

"Me first" is OK!

The third and perhaps most important principle of caught-in-the-middle management states that you simply cannot take care of your organization in the immediate future if you do not first take care of yourself. While the two are mutually dependent, taking care of yourself is primary.

"Taking care of yourself" in the broadest sense means ensuring your well-being in many categories: physical, mental, emotional, financial, spiritual, social, and others. All are relevant, although in this book the emphasis will be on the ones that predominate at work. When we say "taking care of yourself," we mean being sure that your present job does not ruin either your personal life or your long-term career possibilities. Why is this important? Employees, including managers, need periodically to be shown that by working to benefit the organization, they will also benefit themselves. Lacking that, they have little incentive to work, and even less incentive to give extra hours and effort to the organization when needed. In fact, without a clear understanding of the personal rewards available, people who put the organization's needs ahead of their own could actually be acting against their own self-interest. For example, managers may work hard for months to make a merger happen and then find themselves without a job.

The implicit contract between an organization and its employees calls for each to benefit from the other's efforts. When this stops happening, the results can be ugly: the organization treats its people shabbily, or employees begin acting like vultures, tearing the company apart.

These are symptoms of a fundamental misunderstanding of the roles, relationships, and needs of the people involved. Such unhappiness can be avoided if senior management will recognize the simple truth—employees (themselves included) work better when their own welfare is a clear objective of their job.

Caught-in-the-middle management says that neither the personal interest of an employee nor the organizational interest should be satisfied at the expense of the other. To separate them is like saying, "Let's play baseball! Which shall we use, a ball or a bat?" Obviously, both are needed. In applying this analogy to the workplace, we come to the same conclusion. The individual's needs and the organization's needs cannot be separated. Both must be met.

Clearly for that to happen, there must be good faith efforts from everyone involved. But our point is somewhat different. An organization is a group of individuals. For the organization to succeed, those individuals must be cared for. The group's needs will be met most effectively if the group recognizes, abides, and encourages the natural human instincts for self-survival and self-promotion that exist within every individual in the group.

For managers that means not only taking care of themselves, but also realizing that their employees and their superiors all get to do that very same thing — take care of themselves. Only in this way will they be able to take care of the organization.

Surviving and thriving in the middle

The psychoanalyst Erich Fromm pointed out an irony of human beings many years ago. The experience of anxiety makes us seek to remove the cause. The discomfort of anxiety fuels tremendously creative efforts. Those efforts may succeed in removing the anxiety. But in succeeding, we remove the very conditions that fostered our creativity and our ability to manage the anxiety. We remove our success. Fromm's concepts suggest that managers should prefer the middle, and should manage to take care of themselves very well while there.

Caught-in-the-middle management aims at staying in the middle — in the heat, the hurt, and the opportunity. There is almost no opportunity out of the middle. Caught-in-the-middle management aims at taking care of yourself very well in the middle. But the theory does not promise that the fear and pain of being in the middle can be eliminated.

Conclusion

The fear and pain are symptoms of powerful forces, often including the force of change. These forces need to be recognized, respected, and dealt with. When you feel the pain, you will do something about it. You will change yourself. You will change the organization. You will change the factors that determine success.

CHAPTER 2

The next 18 months

At the back of this book is a coupon you can use to order a crystal ball from MGMA. It costs $19.95, and it is guaranteed to have all the answers you need for a successful career in health care. Order yours today!

What? The coupon is missing? Oh, too bad, someone else must have used it already.

OK, OK, we're just having a little fun. There's no coupon, and no crystal ball. (And if there was, do you think you could get it for $19.95?) But as far as predicting what is ahead for your career and for health care, the best you can do is what everyone else is doing. Read everything you can get your hands on. Brainstorm with everyone about how to deal with what is coming. Try to *imagine* the future; try to *create* the future.

Even without a crystal ball, we can tell you this much. Conditions are unusual in health care management today, and they are unusually dangerous for managers. In today's world, any one of a number of external factors can change the entire business landscape for managers, and can change it fast enough to make your head spin. Example: A single act of Congress can upset the most carefully developed five-year business plan. Another example: An insurance-company merger 2,000 miles away can result in big blocks of your patients transferring to other providers.

This chapter advises managers to focus on business and career options that will happen in the next 1 to 18 months, rather than the traditional three to five years. Why? Because change is happening so quickly in our industry that to predict the future any farther out than 18 months (at least to predict it accurately) is nearly impossible.

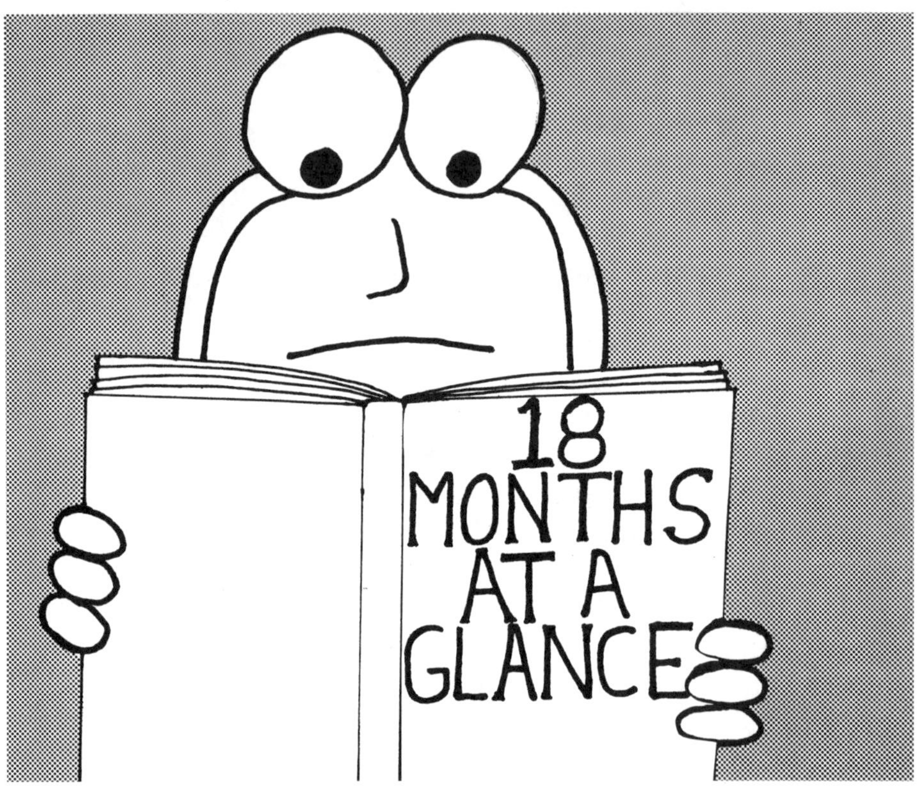

So the next 18 months are the critical period. No matter where you are or how much change has already happened, the next 18 months will bring more change.

Before you start thinking, "No sweat, I can survive anything for 18 months," we need to remind you that this is a "rolling" 18 months. It does not end a year and a half from now, at which time a new period begins. Instead, it is perpetual. It begins anew every month. It's like a high-priced college coach who has a rolling five-year contract. Each year the school has the option of extending the contract a full five years. The coach is always in the first year of a five-year contract — unless the team starts losing too much.

Bad news/good news

The bad news is that one month from now you will be looking forward to another 1-to-18 month period, and talking about that period being the most critical time of your career. The good news is that if you take proper care of yourself and your organization, you will be facing that time period in the best possible shape to succeed.

More troubling news: There will always be insecurity and uncertainty in life and on the job. The bright side is that, in manageable doses, insecurity and uncertainty are not all bad. As Fromm said, one of the ironies of life is that insecurity fuels creativity. As we succeed and become more secure, we tend to lose some creativity. The trick is to keep a balance and to stay in the middle — secure enough to function, but not so secure that we become dull and stale.

The times they are a-changing'

Bob Dylan was right when he first sang that lyric, and he has been right every time he has sung it since then. The times are *always* a-changin'. For American business, times have changed dramatically in recent history. Almost every aspect of the American economy has gone through some form of the reform that is now hitting health care. One big difference: The pace of change itself has increased. In health care we are expected to make changes in two to three years that other industries had 10 or more years to make.

One of the changes is that we can no longer talk about the "American economy." We have to talk about a global economy. Almost anything you buy (including software) now has foreign content or components. Virtually nothing of any complexity is manufactured exclusively in one country, or with parts made only in that country. Many American manufacturers have either gone out of business, or moved all or part of their operations overseas.

Health care is one of the few sectors of our economy that has not been globalized, mainly because it a service industry, and is highly location-dependent. The service must be performed in person, where the patient is.

You might think so, but just consider:

- The latest generation of high-resolution imaging systems can transmit crystal clear X-rays to remote terminals. Is there any reason why a group of radiologists can't sit in their offices in Calcutta and read films shot in Carson City?

  Of course not. So if you manage a radiology practice in Carson City, you could soon be competing for work not only with groups on the other side of town, but also on the other side of the globe;

- What about billing and claims filing? In many practices, those jobs are now being sent by modem to out-of-town clearinghouses for processing. Why not send them beyond our country's borders, if the price and service are right?

- Finally, while it is true that medical services have to be done "in person" with the patient, patients can be moved around a lot more than you might expect. One self-insured plan is now flying cardiac patients to Atlanta from all over the country for certain surgical procedures. Sounds like the plan found a group of cardiologists in Atlanta who wanted the business.

Clues from others

In this country some of the most dramatic change has come in the automobile manufacturing, banking and airlines industries. Nothing in these businesses is as it was five years ago. The American automobile industry has downsized its work force while increasing its productivity and therefore its competitiveness. Huge banking conglomerates have swallowed up hundreds of banks. The airlines, after deregulation, have gone through mergers, bankruptcies, downsizing, layoffs, and hostile takeovers. In each industry phenomenal change is still occurring.

Banking provides a good example. People used to predict that banking would become paperless. In fact, paper is still abundant in banking; the real change is that banks are becoming people-less. Because of competitive pressure, banks have automated their transaction processing to such an extent that they now handle enormously higher transaction volumes with no increase in staff.

This is not to say, "First came the automatic teller, then the automatic doctor." But how about the automatic registration clerk? The automatic "normal lab results" voice-mail machine? (That one is already here.)

The trends that caused these changes in other industries have now caught up with health care. Our "industry" is now being examined by the public. People are asking, "Why medical care costs so much?" and "Why isn't there a better way?" For a long time those of us in health care could fend off such questions by saying, "It's too complicated to explain," or "That's just the way it is," or "We've always done it this way." Those answers don't fly any more.

The rapidity of changes

As health care faces its future, it faces an increased pace of change as a result of four factors: shortened cycles, dynamic technology, challenging attitudes, and new players. These factors are part of why the 18-month perspective makes sense, and these factors are already causing managers to plan and work differently.

Shortened cycles. The industry "change cycle" is shortening in all businesses. Before Japan made the American automobile industry change its behavior, it took as much as five years for a new automobile to go from design to production. Today, this cycle has been shortened in some instances to as short as 18 months.

The same driving force of speed is at work in the delivery of health care. One key area of acceleration is in the way health care is financed. New methods and new alliances are being dreamed up, put in place, or in some cases discarded, at a hectic pace — always in an attempt to stay ahead of the competition. For medical group managers, this means working with shorter time frames against strategic plans that are being continuously revised. The point: These days it seems like all the targets are moving.

Dynamic technology. Cycles have shortened in part because fast-changing technology now allows faster communication of information and faster transportation of goods. These days, even routine documents arrive immediately by fax or E-mail, or overnight by courier. In the medical world, stunning advances in the diagnosis and treatment of illness have taken place during the computer age, creating ever-higher expectations on the part of patients.

A charming recollection: Years ago, when Hollywood got ready to release a new movie, a few prints were sent to a few key cities. Gradually the film made its way to mid-sized and smaller towns. Now the motion picture industry saturates all the population centers at once. Practically all of America can decide on the same day how they like the movie. If it is a children's movie, everyone can have the drinking cups, the dolls, the action figures, the soundtrack CD, and all the other merchandise, even before the movie opens.

In health care much of our information handling is primitive compared to other fields. This situation won't hold up for long. All of us will be expected to take enormous leaps, catching up with the rest of the world in a very short time.

Challenging attitudes. Example: The major parcel delivery services can instantly pinpoint the location of a package anywhere in the country. That's a pretty high standard, but the public is getting accustomed to it. When patients call their physician's office and hear, "Sorry, we can't find your chart," how long will it be before patients get fed up, and go looking for a practice that *can* find the chart? More accurately, they will seek a practice that can find the *information*, because the chart will be in electronic format, not paper.

The implications of these swift changes cannot be summarized by simply saying, "Medical group managers will have to learn how to use the new technology." The technology is the easy part; the real challenge is changing *attitudes*, particularly among physicians.

Attitudes are sometimes very hard to change, particularly under stress and in a short time. In your organization, if the effort to change is not successful, who's head will be on the block — the physician's or the administrator's? We'll give pretty high odds on this bet: it will be the administrator's.

New players. New competitors and investors are entering the market as entrepreneurs, and are hiring health care professionals. Some of these players do not respect tradition and have no personal investment in people and facilities. Most of them have brought ideas from other fields — ideas that are producing rapid and painful change.

In this brave new world, lots of people's lips are saying, "quality of care," but their eyes are saying "profits!" As managers are told to cut costs, increase revenues, raise efficiency and productivity, and "do something about all those capitated patients crowding up the waiting room," managers might face gut-wrenching ethical issues that never existed in the past.

Four change cases

American health care is in the midst of extraordinary change being driven by those who pay for it — both the government and the private business sector. We are going from small independent practices to large integrated systems, from fee-for-service to capitation, and from stable business operations to new and sometimes chaotic methods of doing business.

Group practice decision-making processes are also changing. Authority is being (or will be) delegated to fewer people who are (or will be) empowered to make quick decisions. Otherwise many of our organizations will not survive. And these changes can happen fast. Let's look at a few examples. The companies in the list below are not real, but the cases reflect real situations.

Kirkwood Medical. Kirkwood, a small medical supply company, merged with another company and moved its corporate headquarters. The new company was subsequently acquired by another company in a diversification move. There was little similarity between the old Kirkwood and what it had become 18 months later. Employees had to make hard choices about their careers and their lives as a result.

Coyote Healthcare. While calling itself a system, Coyote was really a large hospital that acquired some smaller hospitals and physicians' practices. Due to a lack of understanding of how medical practices best function, an unanticipated decline in census, and poor planning in general, Coyote became overextended and got into serious financial trouble within 18 months.

Apex Clinic. Apex was a 130-physician group practice that was given a "take it or leave it" offer by a large managed care company. Apex took the deal before they figured out how to handle capitation or control utilization. The bottom fell out within 18 months, when capitation went from 5 to 30 percent of their practice.

MegaHealth. MegaHealth was a new conglomerate of 5 hospitals, 200 physicians, and an insurance partner. It was a giant created out of small pieces, each with a different corporate culture. During its 18-month existence, cultures have clashed, people have fought, market share has decreased, physician income has dropped, and managers have lost jobs. MegaHealth's future is now uncertain.

Possibilities for your organization

What could happen to your organization during the next 18 months? Here are some obvious possibilities.

1. Your organization may go out of business. There will be medical practices and other health care operations that simply close their doors within 18 months. Back to the crystal ball: Wouldn't you want to know if yours is likely to be one that will close?
2. Your organization may be acquired. There are some giants out there who are gobbling up everything in sight.
3. Your organization may acquire other organizations. An acquisition mentality is sweeping health care today. Everybody seems to be buying or selling. If your organization isn't being sold, is it in a position to be buying?
4. Your organization may stagnate. Many medical group managers will be in the same place working for the same organization within 18 months, but the "same" organization may be different by then. As everyone else in the marketplace speeds up, groups (even good groups) that don't keep up will fall behind. This kind of decline is particularly diabolical, because the behavior that made a group successful in the past will simply not bring success in the future.
5. Your organization may grow. There are smart leaders in the health care field who can be counted on to change with the times and be winners.

Possibilities for your career

Here are just a few of the obvious things that could happen to your career during the next 18 months. More will be said about this in chapter four.

1. You may acquire new skills and/or a new career. Many managers are learning new things, and at a rate faster than in the past. We must continue this process, and acquire new skills. New skills are required to compete

in managed care, and to work in the new systems of the future.

Not just new jobs, but new *types* of jobs will develop. These days when you hear someone in medicine talking about "chins," don't assume this is a discussion about the lower part of patient's face. They could be talking about "CHINS," an acronym for "Community Health Information Networks." Unknown a few years ago, CHINS are springing up all over. More to the point, they are creating new types of jobs in the industry. Soon you will be seeing want ads such as:

"CHIN seeks lab interface specialist."

or:

"Fully capitated HMO needs energetic pharmacopia analyst to join expanding team."

These jobs didn't exist before now. But as the financing and delivery systems change, there will be new needs, and new types of jobs created to fill those needs.

2. You may find new business opportunities in health care. The change to managed care and the corporatization of American medicine are creating new niches in the economy. More services will be delivered at patients' homes, for example, as payers continue their efforts to avoid the high cost of inpatient services. Entrepreneurs will rush in to create companies to deliver these services.

3. You may have a new employer. While many of us will be with the same employer in 18 months, many others will not be. Or, you may lose your job and be unemployed.

4. You may work longer hours for the same pay. This is certainly widespread in our field today. People are being asked to worker longer and harder without any added financial incentive.

5. You may or may not take care of yourself. This topic comes up later as an entire chapter. It is relevant to note

now because failure to take care of yourself in this middle period can be devastating to your career.

Conclusion

Changing times can certainly create opportunities. Your goal for the next 18 months should be to create new options for yourself and your organization by acting in your own enlightened self-interest.

Unstable times can also be dangerous. Many things can set your organization on a downward spiral, and that can happen quickly. "Preparedness" is the watchword. Try to anticipate what might be heading your way, and determine how to strengthen yourself and your organization.

In most ways, the managerial talents that have produced success in the past can be relied on to produce success in the future: planning, vision, observation, analysis, dedication, good interpersonal skills, and so on. But the winds of change are at gale force these days, thus even the best managers face risks. How you can cope effectively in this environment is what this book is about. One of the key techniques is to shorten your focus. Pay intense attention to what is likely to happen in the next 18 months. These days, that's where the turning points are to be found.

CHAPTER 3

Develop the worst-case scenario for your organization

Jonathan found himself in a dilemma between semesters in graduate school. Driving home after his final exams, he saw the car's "oil pressure" light blink on for a second. He stopped to check the oil. It was full. He restarted the car, and everything seemed fine for a few minutes. But then the indicator blinked again. Next it started flashing intermittently, and within a short time it was shining steadily, blood-red and insistent.

An engine with no oil pressure is the automotive equivalent of a patient with no blood pressure: it's a critical situation. Jonathan stopped the car and started looking for help.

In the worst case, the car needed an oil-pump transplant, Jonathan reasoned. Best case: The warning light itself was defective.

A mechanic turned the key to the "on" position. Seeing the red glow of the oil-pressure light among all the other indicators, he said, "Well, we know the light works. Must be the pump."

He answered Jonathan's next question without batting an eye, "I'd say about $300 or so."

Jonathan's circumstances complicated the situation. His meager bank balance dictated doing the repair work himself. The weather forecast called for freezing rain followed by a bitter cold snap. "But I'm a smart, resourceful person," he thought. "I'm handy with a tool box. Heck, I'm a graduate student. I can work this out!"

And he did. A farmer friend offered the use of a storage building with a powerful kerosene heater. He bought a rebuilt oil pump for $39.95. Things were looking up. He could get out of this crisis for far less than the price quoted by the mechanic.

Jonathan fired up the kerosene heater and crawled under the car. He settled down into the goo of melted ice, grain chaff and rat droppings, and began the operation. He was uncomfortable but undaunted, and four hours later (with no parts left over!), he started the engine. As it caught, the thought hit him, "Oh my gosh, there were other things that could have caused this problem."

Sure enough, the engine started and purred and burbled happily. But the insolent warning light continued to glow brightly. So the oil pump wasn't the problem at all.

What next? Jonathan went back to the auto parts store and, for $4.75, bought an "oil pressure sending unit." This thumb-sized sensor screws into the side of the engine and controls the warning light. He opened the hood and spent five minutes installing it. That was the problem, and that was the fix. He didn't even have to get under the car.

Cold, wet, dirty, and hungry, he reflected on his use of the worst-case scenario technique. No, that's not right. First, he exercised his vocal cords and his vocabulary. Then he reflected on his use of this method.

Jonathan's instincts for developing a reasonable worst-case scenario were correct. But his methodology had some flaws. Although he had some good luck with the friendly farmer, he also had some bad luck. The mechanic should have suggested checking the sensor before replacing the pump. Jonathan himself didn't know the odds, but any good mechanic will tell you that those little sensors fail much more often than oil pumps do.

Like Jonathan, health care managers today see the warning lights. They feel the urgent need to do something. What they can do is limited by time, abilities, resources, and other factors. Out of practical necessity, managers bet on a chosen course of action, accepting the risk of perhaps fixing the wrong thing, like Jonathan did.

Sometimes, fixing the wrong thing for $44.70 instead of "$300 or so" may not be a bad outcome. Sometimes fixing the wrong thing can be disastrous. The real point is to try to understand the issues and the options before committing to *any* course of action. This chapter describes why and how to develop a reasonable worst-case scenario, and what to do with it once you've got it.

Why develop the worst-case scenario

Patients who feel "What I don't know won't hurt me," and who put off getting tests or treatments, can die from curable diseases. Those patients would benefit from developing a fact-based, worst-case scenario at the earliest warning sign. The idea is to gain knowledge that can lead to action. Obtain as much accurate information as possible in time to act appropriately.

What managers don't know about their organizations can hurt them. Like patients, when circumstances change, managers should develop a fact-based, worst-case scenario for many reasons.

Watch for warning signs.

Any bit of knowledge might require action. Good managers don't ignore warning lights. Instead, they try to find out what is happening, and they try to deal with it. After investigating the situation, a manager might reasonably decide that doing nothing is the best course. Fair enough. But choosing not to investigate at all, to hide one's head in the sand, is poor management, and is asking for trouble.

Issues large and small appear before a manager's eyes every day. Many of these issues are opportunities disguised as problems. Some are time bombs waiting to go off if they are not defused. Examples are easy to come by, and range all the way from "the corporatization of health care" to "the unpredictable actions of government" to "the billing clerk who wants Thursdays off." Issues like these serve to flash warnings for health care managers and their organizations. Managers cannot ignore the signals. Managers must act.

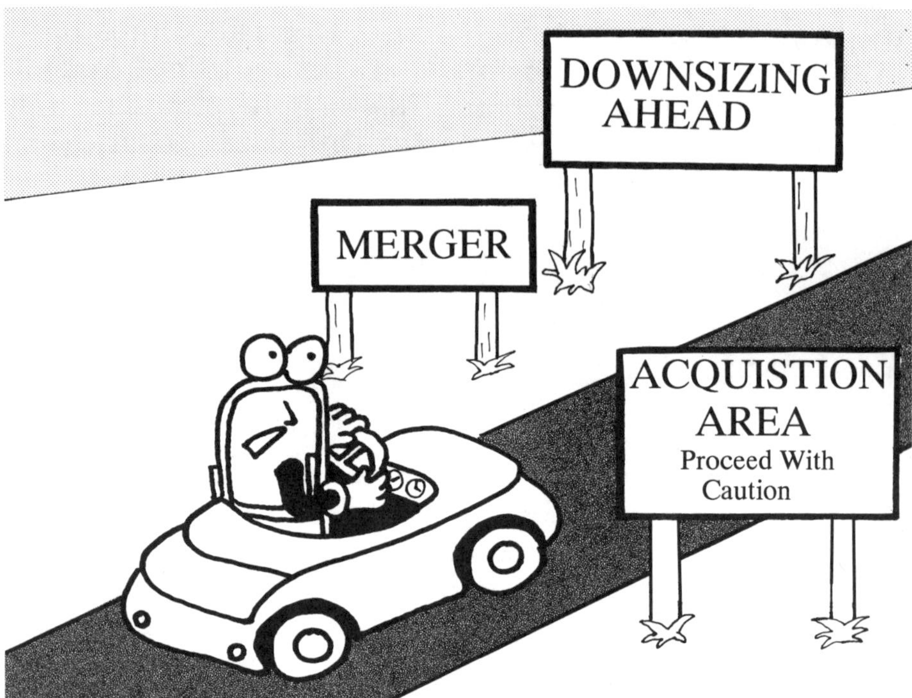

Jonathan had developed the good habit of keeping a wary eye on the dashboard. In a similar fashion, by using the mental discipline needed to develop worst-case scenarios, managers can learn to be constantly on the prowl for knowledge that can be (or should be or must be) turned into action.

Get good information.

If knowledge sometimes requires action, effective action depends on the most complete and accurate information that can be obtained. Getting good information is part and parcel of doing a worst-case scenario.

This is the area where Jonathan's technique was faulty. He didn't ask enough questions, didn't solicit enough opinions, didn't investigate all the options. He didn't get the facts, so the facts got him. If he had done a better job gathering and interpreting information, he might have been back on the road soon after he first noticed the problem.

In the story above, Jonathan's options depended on a number of factors. If he owned another car, immediate action might not have been critical. If he had plenty of money, he might reject the option of fixing the car himself. If he had a week of free time, he might wait until the weather improved. Regardless, the sooner he got the most complete and accurate information that could be obtained, the sooner he would know his options and the more effectively he could act.

Set yourself up for nice surprises.

You want your surprises to be nice. Although it was nice for Jonathan to avoid having to spend $300, he still spent nearly 10 times as much as was actually needed. He also had to endure some real discomfort and anxiety. Think of how much nicer the story would have been if he had barely gotten his hands dirty, and had spent only $5, and gotten back on the road in five minutes. That would have been the outcome if he'd done a bit more brainwork.

The irony in this story, of course, is that Jonathan could have safely ignored the warning light, and in all likelihood nothing bad would have happened. After all, the oil pressure inside the engine was perfectly fine all along. The difficulties were caused by a mistaken *indicator,* by an erroneous *reading* of the oil pressure.

So, is this story a poor example to use? After all, it really didn't matter whether Jonathan did a worst-case analysis. It didn't even matter whether he acted or not.

No, this is not a bad example. It's a wonderful example, because it is so true-to-life. Sometimes ignorance *is* bliss. Sometimes fate smiles on you no matter what, and you can't make a mistake even if you try. On the other hand, sometimes you get completely clobbered no matter how well you prepare.

The real point: Managers who depend on the best case

are setting themselves up for failure when a less-than-best case occurs. Managers who develop an effective plan for taking care of themselves and their organizations in the *worst* case are setting themselves up for success and nice surprises.

How to develop the worst-case scenario

A "worst-case scenario" is not a description of the most horrible thing that could possibly happen. After all, if an errant comet wipes out all life on earth your difficulties at work become moot. Therefore, your plans will not normally need to make provisions for errant comets. Instead, the worst-case scenario defines the most difficult and costly issues you might *reasonably* need to manage, given the uncertainties of the situation.

"Uncertainties" is a key word, because what we are talking about involves predicting the future — always a risky proposition. But the best way to predict the future is to create the future, and to create the future you must start with a plan. So your worst-case scenario should look like it came from the Planning Committee, not the Ouija Board.

In fact, the picture you prepare of the worst case should actually *be* a strategic plan or an operational plan — one of a number of plans you have in the works at a given moment. The worst-case scenario will be the most pessimistic of the plans, but accurate and workable nonetheless.

An example: Let's say you are planning a big wedding reception for a Saturday in June. You will want the reception to be outdoors, in your lovely formal garden, just when the lilacs and azaleas and irises will be so completely stunning. But if it rains, you'd better have *someplace else* to put those 400 hungry, unforgiving guests.

In other words, we need at the minimum to develop "Plan A" (the achingly-beautiful-perfect-day-in-June plan), and "Plan B" (a cold-wet-windy-dreary-I-can't-believe-this-is-happening-to-us! plan). Plan B is your "worst-case scenario" regarding weather.

Here are some techniques that help when developing the worst-case scenario.

Get to know the issues, including "soft" issues.

Gathering relevant and objective data about the situation is a critical step. But in addition, managers have to recognize the fact that challenges can produce anxieties and fears in everyone involved. It is a mistake to ignore those feelings. Treat them as teachers who have much to tell you about yourself and the other people involved.

For instance, Jonathan's immediate response to the engine's warning sign was mild panic:

> "Ohmygoshmycarisdyingandidonthaveenough
> moneyforanotheronesoIwillhavetodropoutofgra
> duateschoolandIcantdoanythingtoearnalivings
> oIllprobalblybehomelesscoldandhungrybynext
> ChristmasandIwillneverbesuccessful!"

His was a fairly normal reaction, and one that took awhile to subside before he could think more clearly. That same phenomenon occurs on an organizational scale. Managers must realize that people and organizations go through a *process* made up of many steps when dealing with major challenges. The process itself is an issue to be studied.

Project the current situation into the future.

Here's a simple example of making a useful projection. Jean, the manager of a large group practice in a market that was rapidly moving toward capitation, conducted a financial analysis that showed:

1. Revenue grew over the past five years, but the rate of growth had declined steadily;

2. Expenses (as a percentage of revenues) were on the increase; and

3. If these trends continued, the group would be running in the red in four years.

The physicians weren't happy to hear this, but the numbers didn't lie.

There are many approaches that might be taken to reverse the trends, but the point is: Jean's habit of projecting the current situation into the future had the very beneficial effect of letting the group deal with the issues while their heads were still well above water.

Remove each assumption underlying the current situation and examine the consequences of removing it.

For example, remove fee-for-service and replace it with varying degrees of capitation. Graph the effects on revenue, expenses, and profits. Then ask other questions. What investments are required? How does patient care change? How do administrative staff responsibilities change? How much money will be available for salaries? What will happen to staffing levels? Can the organization afford its own billing operation? Continue asking questions until you understand the implications of this one changed assumption.

Now remove the assumption about the number of patients. What if the number remains stable? What if it grows five percent a year? What if it decreases by five percent instead? Compute and graph the revenue, expenses and profits, and ask the same questions about the organization.

This exercise focuses attention on the critical success factors. It identifies the areas where change must occur if you are to take care of your organization. Absent success on these factors, other questions about the organization become moot.

Identify and examine new assumptions.

Health care literature in the early 1990's proclaimed that governmental action would cause major restructuring of our industry. By mid-decade the government efforts had floundered.

So the people who said the government would cause upheaval in our industry were wrong, right? Well, yes and no. They got the part wrong about who was going to cause the restructuring. As it turns out, the private sector instead of the government has triggered the changes. But they sure got it right that big changes were heading our way.

But the real lesson is that a new assumption ("private sector pressure") was just crying to be plugged in to the scenario. When you are preparing business plans, including worst-case scenarios, it is *always* a good idea to look for new elements that might affect your projections.

How to start

The previous four steps are one way to approach the task of analyzing what your organization may face in the future. Other techniques abound, but the conceptual framework is always the same. Gather facts and opinions. Try to ask the questions whose answers will lead your organization to a successful future.

All good managers eventually discover that it is easier to *avoid* trouble than it is to get out of trouble once you are there. The kind of analysis that this chapter recommends can be a big help in keeping your business out of trouble. And when you do this for your organization, you can also develop a wealth of very important information that applies to your own career.

Often when you are doing analyses you will not have perfectly accurate or complete information. Act on what you have. Make assumptions when you need to, using national figures or other reasonable estimates. Then keep track of your assumptions. Also note how much confidence you have in your projections. The real point: Just start.

Conclusion

Developing a worst-case scenario produces the best information available at the time. It gives the kind of information Jonathan had: incomplete and imperfect, but the best available. It's the kind of information caught-in-the-middle managers always have: incomplete and imperfect, but the information on which they must act to take care of themselves and their organizations.

CHAPTER 4

Develop the worst-case scenario for your career

Once you've developed the worst-case scenario for your organization, you then need to develop one for your career. Given what you see as the possible future for the organization, ask, "What does it mean for me?"

Unfortunately, some people who can easily develop a worst-case scenario for their organization are unable to do the same thing for their career. Some see only disaster and doom, while others believe "It could not happen to me." Reality tells us that most people should see themselves caught in the middle between these two extremes, at varying stages of risk to their careers.

There are two reasons why so many people have difficulty in developing a realistic worst-case scenario for their career. First, some people feel guilty because they view this exercise as an act of disloyalty. Second, there is a real fear associated with this process. We will discuss these two roadblocks before outlining techniques for developing the worst-case scenario for your career.

Loyalty ain't what it used to be

Loyalty today is more transitional than it was in previous decades. It's a simple fact that the economy is changing so fast that there is no "status quo," and organizations have much less loyalty for their employees. Large companies lay off thousands of workers or move entire plants out of the country in pursuit of cheap labor. Moves that appear disloyal to the employee are labeled as necessary for survival by management. On the flip side of the coin, old-time fans are appalled when professional athletes change teams after nearly every season, selling their services to the highest bidder. Similarly, employees change companies at the drop of a hat.

In medical group management, and in the rapidly changing health care field, loyalty is starting to take a beating in your locale. Looking out for yourself is necessary and appropriate. If you don't, nobody else will. Be as loyal as your organization deserves, and be loyal to your staff, but keep your eyes open so that you can be loyal intelligently.

Furthermore, to do a good job evaluating your own career, you first have to take a hard look at some important aspects of your organization. This kind of analysis is critical to the success of any business. So, far from being an act of disloyalty, this exercise may have specific benefits for your organization, if it is wise enough to use them.

The only thing we have to fear...

The other factor that keeps people from doing a worst-case scenario is fear. Many people live in fear of the future, preferring not to face it. Fear causes some people to become paralyzed and others to become hostile. A decision made out of fear is not likely to be the best decision you can make.

Your goal is not to eliminate fear, but instead to manage it. The person who understands and manages fear can be effective. Ask yourself, "What is it I fear? Is it death, unemployment, loss of status, divorce, desertion, ostracism, illness, bankruptcy, lack of sufficient funds for retirement, being forced to retire, being disabled, getting old...?" (Quite an inventory!) Get your fears out and look at them. Force yourself to think about each one until they no longer cause you stress.

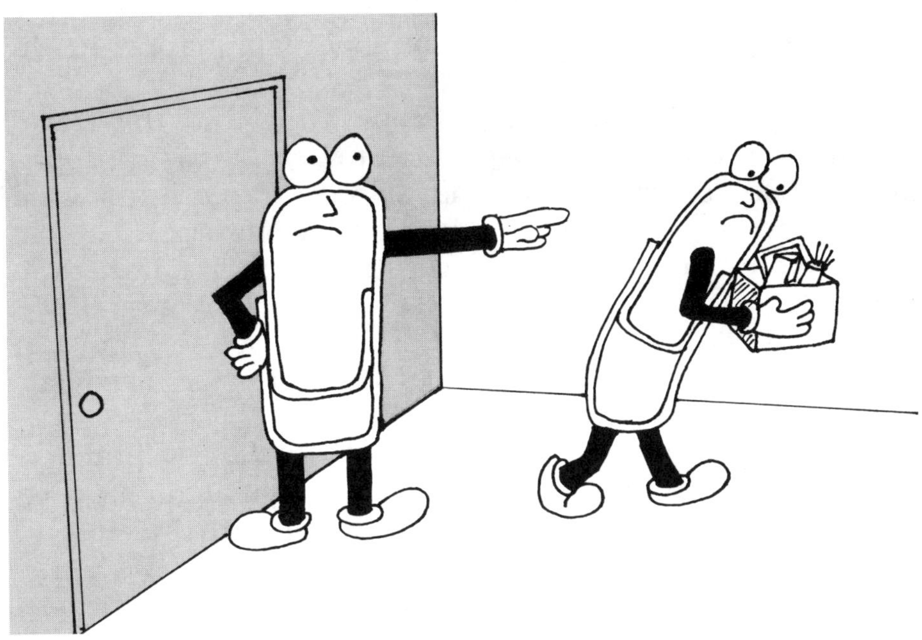

How to develop the worst-case scenario for your career

Let's now make a list of techniques for developing the worst-case scenario for your career.

Keep perspective.

Stress can diminish your peripheral vision. Under stress many managers tend to lose the ability to see the big picture. It's as if they are in a large room with their nose against the wall, and their eyes focused on the wallpaper. Get your nose away from the wall!

Some managers have developed self-protective warning systems. When stress gets too high, an internal alarm goes off and says, "OK, it's time to get out of here and go work in my garden" (or go fishing, go shopping, go get a massage...whatever works to reduce stress).

However, many managers don't have such warning systems. They burrow their noses into the wall until their eyeballs are touching the wallpaper. This is not a recommended position from which to see the pattern of the wallpaper, much less anything actually happening in the room.

Until you see the room, the building and the world beyond, you are not in any position to develop an appropriate worst-case scenario for your career. From a distorted perspective your thoughts run to extremes such as "I'm going to die," or "I'm about to get fired," or "I'll tell them to take this job and shove it!" These feelings may actually fit into an appropriate worst-case scenario, but you have to be calm, cool, collected, and objective to develop a realistic picture that will do you any good.

Dan, the administrator for a large cardiology practice, was in his office just before noon one day catching up on some paperwork when Scott, his Appointment and Registration Manager, walked in and said, "Can we talk?" Dan prided himself on always being available to his people. So he laid his paperwork aside and said, "Of course, what's on your mind?"

One look at Scott told Dan a lot. Scott was a nervous person who took great pride in his work and wanted everything to be perfect every day. Dan had never been able to convince Scott that perfection is not a realistic business goal in running a physician's office. Sure the physicians want perfection, but Dan had learned the hard way that it would never happen. Dan understood that on any given day things go wrong. His job, and Scott's, was to anticipate and eliminate as many mistakes as possible, then fix things that got broken.

Scott felt personally responsible for every problem. When a physician snapped at him, he felt he was truly to blame. His self-punishing attitude made his blood pressure go up. Dan had talked to Scott about this on numerous occasions, but he had never been able to break through Scott's defenses.

Today Dan decided to take a different tack when Scott started telling him about a whole series of little problems that had been nibbling on him all morning. Dan said, "I don't want to talk about those heartburns." He leaned across the desk, looked at Scott and said, "Back up away from the wall and look at the room. You're focusing on one little corner of the room and not on the big picture."

It took a few minutes for Scott to grasp the analogy and to understand what Dan was saying. Each time Scott wanted to talk about a specific, Dan made him focus on the broader issues. Each time Scott expressed anger at someone or something that wasn't going right, Dan agreed that it probably wasn't right but added, "Scott, it will never be perfect."

After a half hour or so of Scott venting and Dan helping him focus on the broader issues, Dan ordered Scott to turn in his beeper, and go away until he gained perspective. Dan told him, "I don't care where you go, but get out of here and relax. Don't think about this place or your job until you are sure your blood pressure is down and you feel no stress. At that point if you have constructive ideas about how to make the work flow better, or how to organize your duties better, or how to improve the big picture, jot them down and we'll talk about them when you get back."

Scott argued, saying he couldn't get away because his being out would only cause things to get worse. No one would do his work and it would just pile up. Dan replied, "If you kill yourself on this job, you won't be here to do it. So we might as well start learning how to address your absence now rather than later."

Finally Scott agreed, turned over his beeper, and left Dan's office. He went back to his office to tell his subordinates that he was leaving. People started running up to him with questions and complaints. At first he tried to address them, but then, remembering what Dan had said, he simply walked out. He went home, changed clothes, went for a long walk. That night he took his family to a movie.

The next morning he called Dan and said, "I'll probably be back tomorrow." Dan reminded him not to come back until he had made a list, developed in a stress-free setting, of things to be done to make the situation better. That day Scott went to the river and watched the water for hours. Finally a thought hit him, then another and another. He came home with three pages of notes.

He went back to work the next day, reviewed his list with Dan, and started functioning just a little differently. One of the items on his list was to stop letting people dump every problem in his lap. He would learn to say "No." He learned to say:

"No, sorry, I can't talk now. See me after lunch."

"No, it would be better if *you* made that phone call."

"No, you talk to her about that and work it out. If you can't, then both of you come to see me."

In gaining perspective, Scott had taken the first step towards developing the worst-case scenario for his career.

Remember the difference in CAE and CEE.

Philip Beard, a well-known health care consultant, tells a story about a participant in a seminar coming up to him and saying, "You forgot to mention CAE and CEE." Not being familiar with these terms, Beard asked for clarification.

The response was "CAE is a Career-Altering Event and CEE is a Career-Ending Event."

Clearly your task in developing a worst-case scenario is to plan for Career-Altering Events and to avoid Career-Ending Events. How do you tell the difference? One way is to check what your organization is doing compared with the rest of the industry. If your employer says, "I'll never take capitation," or "We don't need to be part of a network," or "Things will work out," look out, you may be heading for a CEE!

Figure out what will happen if things turn sour.

If your worst-case scenario for the organization indicates that things may go bad, what are your chances for survival? A healthy dose of "What happens to me?" is vital. If it looks like the organization will survive, who will likely be left? If your organization appears to be in trouble, will it likely be acquired or just close up?

Tom was a highly skilled top-down manager who had spent 22 years running larger and larger hospitals. One day he was put in charge of three physician practices acquired by his organization, Coyote Healthcare. (Coyote was called a health care delivery system, but it really was a big hospital that owned some smaller hospitals, and now owned three physician groups.) Tom was told to "Take charge, run those offices, implement economies of scale, increase productivity and lower costs."

Any surprise that disaster occurred and that Tom was in the job market within a year? Not a good place for a 55-year-old these days. Tom hadn't developed the worst-case scenario for his organization in advance of being given this assignment. Without that, he had no reason to develop a worst-case scenario for his career.

He didn't think through the possibilities. For example, Coyote might not be able to run the physicians' offices better than the medical group managers who had been doing it. He did not think about the physicians' loss of commitment to an organization that they no longer owned. Worst of all, he did not reflect on "What happens to me if this whole thing turns sour?"

Should I stay or go?

This step is a doozey. You must ask yourself the question, "If things continue on this way, should I stay or go?" You must be honest with yourself, look fear in the eye, and make a preliminary decision to stay or go — to keep plugging or resign.

Your decision is preliminary and you shouldn't act on it, but just note it and set a date to review it. This decision frees you to concentrate your energies on taking care of yourself and your organization. Remember, you can't take care of your organization if you don't take care of yourself.

It is true that reality looks different to objective people in the same situation. Nonetheless, you must be as honest as you can with yourself. You may be wrong in some of your perceptions, but the idea is to describe the situation to yourself as honestly as you can. Without an honest appraisal of your organization, the environment, and your spot in it, you cannot make a truly informed decision.

We know a former commissioner of a state Department of Health who was talking to his assistant about what he wanted to accomplish in the next year. His assistant reminded the commissioner that there recently had been an election, and that one of the incoming governor's key advisors was a person the commissioner had once fired.

This didn't raise the commissioner's defenses. The assistant then said, "Have you noticed that your phone doesn't ring much any more and no one comes to see you?" The commissioner acknowledged this state of affairs. The assistant then made his point, "Boss, you're the only person in town who doesn't realize that you're a lame duck!"

The commissioner got the point, but a little late. In three weeks he was unemployed. He had been lying to himself for months rather than being honest and making plans accordingly.

To tell yourself the truth, sit down at your computer, or sit down with pencil and paper, and in two columns list the reasons to stay and the reasons to go. Putting the cold, hard facts on paper brings a feeling of reality.

Sometimes you will be surprised at the list, and one side will have many more entries than the other. Other times it comes out to be more equal. In either case, you're better off than your peers who don't regularly conduct this exercise.

By the way, this is not easy to do. In fact it's downright hard, and even painful. It's much easier to lie to yourself if you keep the issues in your head instead of committing them to paper.

Do a reality check.

Having gained perspective, having thought about whether you are facing a Career-Altering Event or a Career-Ending Event, having figured out what will probably happen to you if things turn sour, and having made a preliminary decision to stay or go, you now want to do a reality check with management. You need to find out if they understand the issues, and how and whether they might respond as things change for the organization.

You can do this by developing a "plan" for your part of the organization, and taking it to management. Call it a trial balloon. Although you have your own purpose for presenting it, the plan must absolutely be a legitimate proposal to deal with a current or expected business need. Why? Because there is always the possibility your plan will be approved, and you will actually have to implement it!

Still, your goal in presenting the plan is not to get it immediately accepted, but rather to gauge the reaction of management. You want to know if management understands its own situation, and if it is preparing for the changes you see coming. You also want to know how much support and involvement upper management is willing to give you and others at your level of the organization.

This, of course, has to be a plan appropriate for your level of the organization. If you are responsible for paticnt registration, your plan will need to show how to manage issues of patient registration to improve current operations and prevent the worst-case scenario for the organization. If you are responsible for a satellite clinic, your plan may deal with how to improve services at that satellite, how to attract more patients, or how to ensure appropriate utilization of services by capitated patients. In Medical Records, you may want to work on electronic medical records. In Occupational Medicine, you might propose direct contracts with industry.

The plan should not go into great detail. Again, the object is not necessarily to get approval, but instead to test your superiors' understanding of the issues, and to gauge their willingness to act. If top management understands the issues and encourages action, there will be ample opportunities to develop a comprehensive plan.

What did they say? Do they understand?

After presenting a plan to address something you think needs attention in one of your area responsibilities, listen carefully and objectively to the reactions. The reactions tell you how your organization will function in light of the worst-case scenario which you have constructed for your organization. Their responses will answer these questions about your organization:

- Does top management understand the trends in health care today?
- Will management empower you and others to act for the good of the organization?
- Can you obtain enough information to make informed judgments about the future of the organization?
- Are the core values of the organization consistent enough with your values for you to invest the time and effort to avoid or survive the worst case?

These questions confirm or revise the conclusions you made about your superiors. Consider a "No" answer to any of these questions a warning sign of a potential CAE or CEE.

Add up the numbers.

If you like to quantify things, you will like this method of computing a mathematical value for your organization in relation to the environment in which it exists. Here's the formula:

THE ENVIRONMENT + MANAGEMENT'S REACTION = YOUR DECISION

First, here's the scale for rating the environment:

5. This place is the big winner in health care;
4. Things look pretty good;
3. It's about 50/50 whether this place survives another 3 years;
2. Things look bad; or
1. We won't make it through the fiscal year.

And here is the scale for rating the reaction of management:

5. Enthusiastic support. "Wow, why didn't I think of that!" "How soon can you start on it?" "What do you need?";
4. Mildly supportive. "Hmmmmm." "Maybe." "Let's get together on this next week";
3. Don't care. "Oh, things will work out";
2. Mildly annoyed. "Who told you to work on that?"; or
1. Openly hostile. "Don't let the door hit you on the way out."

Add your organization's score from the first list, and management's score from the second list. In this highly scientific model, you need a score of six or better to feel like you should stay.

A score above six means either that things don't look bad or that management's reaction to your ideas was positive — or both. A score below six means that you may want to change your preliminary decision or at least shorten the time until your next review.

A good score should not sway you too far; consider it an opportunity for more dialogue and further investigation. Likewise, a low score does not mean you should leave the organization. It does mean that you must place blind trust in management as long as you stay there, and it does mean you should carefully and frequently look for additional warning signs.

Check it out.

When Jonathan dealt with his oil pump in the previous chapter, he verified his worst-case scenario. But he verified it with a person whose knowledge was not appropriate for the task. Neither the mechanic nor Jonathan lacked intelligence or logic, but it must also be said that neither one had the factual foundation for an accurate diagnosis.

Jonathan said, "It must be the gauge or the oil pump, right?" The mechanic agreed. The terms of the question limited the possible answers, as demonstrated by the eventual discovery that it was neither of those components, but something entirely different — something they had not thought about.

You must verify your observations, your analyses, and your conclusions. Proper verification includes reviews by knowledgeable, open-minded individuals who will challenge the assumptions that lie under your questions. Verify your work with several competent individuals. Ask them to spell out *their* assumptions. Each time be sure that you are both dealing with the same scenario.

Verify with objective people who act as advocates for your well-being and who keep confidences. These criteria eliminate family members, co-workers, and competitors.

Review your preliminary decision to stay or go.

When the date you set arrives, make one of three decisions:

1. Stay for another 1-18 months if the circumstances continue;

2. Leave within 1-18 months if the circumstances continue; or

3. Leave as soon as possible, doing the best that you can for the organization in the interim.

Making preliminary decisions and confirming them at a set date helps offset the negative effects of incomplete and imperfect information. There's no secret to it. Simply select a date and define the standards by which you will decide. For example, "If we do not begin preparing for capitation by mm/dd/yy, I will stay no more than six months, unless new information suggests other standards and/or a different date."

The way you stay or go is important. You don't want to make an uninformed decision to stay *or* to go; you don't want to stay or go out of fear; and you don't want to be ineffective in any case. If you go, you don't want to burn your bridges. Behave ethically and honestly, do your work well, and encourage your people to do the same.

Conclusion

Developing the worst-case scenario is not the act of a pessimist or the result of negative thinking. It is instead an act of courage and objectivity, and it is critically important to taking care of yourself and safeguarding your career.

CHAPTER 5

Take care of yourself

Chapter 5–Take care of yourself

Stated simply, this chapter takes the position that managers must pay more attention to themselves and to their own needs. Commitment to an organization is important — if the organization deserves commitment — but commitment to yourself should be primary. If you don't take care of yourself, you can't take care of your organization.

We will try to show you how to balance your commitment to the organization with its commitment to you. We will discuss the warning signs of problems in an organization. We will discuss how to heed the warning signs, and we'll offer guidance on how to act on them. But first we will tell you about Tim.

"Toto, I have a feeling we're not in Kansas anymore"

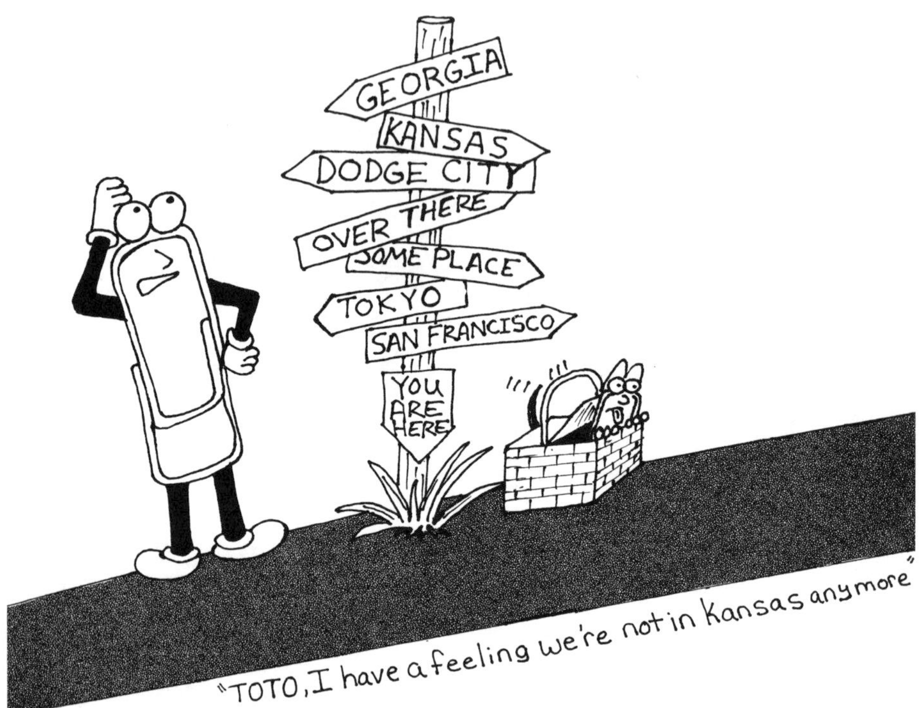

In "The Wizard of Oz" Dorothy wasn't talking about corporate transfers, but Tim could relate to her concern. One difference was that while Dorothy wanted to be in Kansas, Tim was there but didn't want to be. He was unemployed in Kansas and didn't want to be unemployed *or* in Kansas.

How Tim got to Kansas and became unemployed is our case study in "How Not to Take Care of Yourself."

Tim had been the Personnel Department Director of Kirkwood Medical, a medium-sized health supply company in Georgia. Kirkwood was an 18-year-old, family-owned business. Tim had been with Kirkwood for 15 of those years and had seen it grow tenfold over that time. He viewed Kirkwood as a good employer and looked forward to a long association.

One morning Tim opened the newspaper to a headline that screamed "TIM — YOU'RE MOVING TO KANSAS!"

(That's not really what it said, but that's what it meant to Tim.) His company had announced a merger with another company, located in Kansas.

Tim's position was not high enough in the company for him to have been informed in advance about the merger plans. And once the deal was struck, the company foolishly gave the information to the news media before notifying employees at every level. As a result, Tim was caught completely by surprise.

He did not reflect on his situation; he did not consider any option. He just assumed that he should stay with his company and go to Kansas, if they gave him the choice. They did and he did, and he was grateful. He thought that his job in Georgia had been secure and he assumed that it would be the same in Kansas. He wasn't tuned in to any of the warning signs that were available, either before or after the move. (We'll deal with warning signs a little later.)

Tim didn't explore options, he just moved to Kansas! He was now with a bigger company and had bigger responsibilities. It was his job to merge people from two completely different organizations and cultures into a new, integrated unit.

Kirkwood had been a top-down managed company; the new one, Jones Supply, had used a more participatory management style. Grateful that the company had kept him, he threw himself into the difficult process of helping to create the personnel department of the new company. It was a really hard year for Tim. The Jones people did not believe in telling people what to do. They wanted to know what he thought and expected him to take ownership and make decisions.

Tim more than survived the process. He involved people, made decisions, and managed a smooth and successful transition. Some people lost their jobs, but Tim handled his part compassionately, and felt good about himself and what he had achieved. Over that year he worked harder, and put in longer hours than he ever had before. He thought he had grown professionally, and that Kansas wasn't too bad.

Guess what! One morning his newspaper informed him that another merger had taken place and the new headquarters would be at the home office of Mammoth Supply, in Maryland. His first reaction was "I hope I don't have to move again."

He got his wish; there was no job for him in Maryland. Tim was devastated. He had been caught by surprise again. He felt totally helpless. He had been too absorbed in his work to heed the warning signs. As details became known, it was announced that the Personnel Director in Maryland would head the new combined unit. She didn't see a place for Tim.

He had moved cross country to a strange town out of total loyalty to his company, which now (if ever) had no loyalty to him. Now he was unemployed. He wasn't unemployed back where he came from, where he knew some people and could put out feelers for a job, but instead he was unemployed in a strange town.

What happened to Tim can happen to any manager caught in the middle. Practicing caught-in-the-middle management might help, because one of the mainstays of this philosophy is knowing how to take care of yourself.

A really happy ending to Tim's story could be that after he lost his job, he was forced to take charge of his future. He eliminated all the "circumstances beyond his control," and through pluck and luck got a great new job or even a new career, made millions, and found happiness and success.

The point: Why did Tim have to be "forced to take charge of his future?" What was stopping him from doing that *before* he lost his job?

Warning signs

Let's not dwell on the outcome of Tim's situation right now. Instead, let's look at warning signs and then at the things that Tim didn't do to take care of himself throughout this process. Let's answer these questions: What are warning signs? What do they look like? Is there a list of them?

What are warning signs?

Warning signs are signals that something has changed or that something is about to change. Every such signal isn't a warning sign, but every such signal needs to be treated as a potential warning sign. If you don't notice the signs or even know how to look for them, you may be in serious trouble already. It is not overly dramatic to say that everybody in health care today should be looking for warning signs.

You can recognize a warning sign easily: something is different. There are all kinds of bosses and all kinds of organizations, but when something changes, there must be a reason.

There are even warning signs that there will be warning signs. Any driver has seen such signs as "Stop Sign Ahead." It's a warning sign to look for the warning sign. There were some big ones out there that Tim missed: changes in the health care market, changes in reimbursement policy, and the attention that health care reform was getting in the press. Tim didn't buy the premise that change was coming. He was, therefore, oblivious to the signs in front of him for months before his career fell apart.

If you notice one warning sign, file it for reference. If you see two or three, check them out. Here are some of the more common ones that Tim might have seen if he had been looking — if he had heeded the first sign that said "Warning Signs Ahead":

- Some bits and pieces in the press that show change: Stock prices rise or fall dramatically; merger plans are announced; a shake-up in your organization or in a competitor's organization is reported;

- All of the sudden you're out of the loop: People who used to talk to you, now don't have much to say, and they don't involve you in things;

- There's a major flurry of activity: All of a sudden they're painting everything. Could it be they're getting ready to sell it?;

- People are coming and/or going: Trips and meetings are scheduled a lot more than usual;

- There are unexplained strangers in your midst: Visitors appear frequently for closed-door conferences;

- There's a decline in maintenance, or supplies are harder to get: Could it be money trouble?;

- There's a lack of response from the bosses to a memo about a subject that in the past would have gotten results: The bosses seem preoccupied. People aren't asking you for the kinds of things they asked you for in the past; or

- People are asking you for all kinds of analyses about employees, contracts, etc.: Why is there such a need for these specifics?

What do warning signs look like?

Warning signs are like the old joke about the religious fellow caught in a flood. His neighbors came for him in a boat, but he refused to leave, saying, "The Lord will take care of me." As the water reached the second floor, the National Guard came in a bigger boat, but he refused to leave, saying, "The Lord will take care of me."

By the time the National Guard returned in a helicopter, he was on the roof with the water lapping at his heels. But again he refused to leave, and he repeated his statement that the Lord would take care of him.

He drowned and went to heaven, where he confronted St. Peter by saying, "Why wasn't I saved?" St. Peter peered over his glasses and said, "We sent two boats and a helicopter. What more did you want?"

Tim may have been like this fellow. The warning signs were there. Some warning signs are obvious and some are subtle. They may or may not be accompanied by thunder and lightning.

Is there a helpful list?

The previous list contains some of the more obvious signs, and with a little imaginative observation you could add many items to that list. Here are a few other signs Tim missed:

- Kirkwood Supply lost out on a bid to be a major supplier to a new hospital company that bought five area hospitals — all former customers of Kirkwood;
- The CEO rather suddenly "moved up" to become Chairman of the Board. The new CEO was half his age and full of new ideas; and
- Top management people started making frequent trips to Kansas; and
- Some of Tim's peers were "looking around at other opportunities."

What if Tim had heeded the signs? Could he have done something? That depends on how early in the game he took notice of change, and on how willing he was to do something. There are things Tim should have done, that all of us should do, with or without warning signs. They fall under the heading of "How to Take Care of Yourself."

How to take care of yourself

Obviously, taking care of yourself is not something you do only once. It is a process, a habit, perhaps even a way of living, and it must be ongoing.

This book is about your life at work. There are many other aspects of life where the advice "take care of yourself" could apply, including financial, physical, social, emotional, and spiritual areas. Those are equally important but not within the domain of this book. However, their interconnectedness and their influence on your life at work must be recognized.

What are the things that people need to do to take care of themselves? Here's a list. It is not exhaustive, but simply pinpoints some of the things that have helped many people find success:

- Reflect;
- Develop new skills;
- Develop alternatives;
- Build and maintain a network;
- Read;
- Watch trends; and
- Keep your résumé current.

Let's briefly examine each one.

Reflect

It is amazing that a notion this fundamental is so widely ignored. Time spent in reflection is hardly ever wasted. Set aside time each week for reflecting on yourself and your organization, and on how they interact. Think about what you want to achieve. Make plans. Consider alternatives. Ponder and wonder. Think.

Remember, the major limiting factor for options is inside each individual. You only have the options that you are willing to consider.

Develop new skills

Tim had devoted most of his career to Kirkwood's Personnel Department. He knew the personnel software

Kirkwood used on an outdated mainframe, but he hadn't kept up with developments in modern systems. He wasn't very adaptable. He only knew his company and his piece of the business.

Tim had a co-worker at Kirkwood named Lynn who had a different approach to her career. Lynn was in charge of shipping and receiving. She had been shocked when she heard Dr. C. Everett Koop say in 1991 that health care was going to crash and burn in the 1990's like the airlines and the savings and loans did in the 1980's.

Lynn decided to make herself more valuable to her employer or to future employers by developing new skills. No one told her to do it; she just did it. She learned how to use computers and became proficient in computer programs for word processing, financial and personnel management, and in-house publishing.

She tried to upgrade the tracking system in central supply but her boss didn't see the need. Not to be deterred, Lynn developed plans for what should be done. After the merger, her new boss was impressed that she had a lot to offer, and gave her a choice of several attractive jobs. Lynn had made herself more valuable and had gained more options because she had actively worked to develop new skills.

Develop some alternatives

Develop some alternate ways to get money while you're looking for a job if you become unemployed. There's nothing wrong, and everything right, with developing a side-line skill. Dan, Kirkwood's MIS Director, had developed some options and did not have to move. Part of the reason that he had developed alternatives was that he had been burned years before and he had decided that he would not be caught off guard again. He had gone through a period of unemployment and had been forced to develop options then. As a result, he had finished his Master's Degree, which had enabled him to renew his high school teaching certificate. He also got a real estate license.

Dan viewed these two pieces of paper as his safety net if he ever got fired again. He felt sure he would be able at least to be a substitute teacher and to work with a friend's real estate firm while looking around for another "permanent" position.

Build and maintain a network

It is important to have a network, so you're plugged in with the widest possible assortment of contacts. You help people and they help you. If you lose your job, your network is the place where you'd go to start your search. Networking is about relationships — relationships of trust with people who share your interests and have some concern for you.

Even if Tim had wanted to talk over his "options" before moving to Kansas, he didn't have many people to talk with. His network in Georgia had been fairly limited and consisted mostly of his family and a few people he worked with. He really hadn't reached out to develop a broader network. Tim didn't see much need for networking, and felt he was far too busy at his job to spend the time required.

Linda, the Assistant to the CEO of the Georgia company, was different. She was married to the owner of five fast food outlets, and she was a third-generation resident of the community. She had lots of family and friends in the area. She had one child in the eighth grade and one who was a sophomore in high school.

When the Kirkwood merger came, she didn't even think about moving. She had seen the warning signs months before and had started discreetly calling some of her most trustworthy and well-placed contacts. You can bet that she was situated before the news officially hit.

Read

Managers have so much material to read that many of them get burned out on reading. Many managers get to the point that they can't read for fun, or to help themselves. But as a manager, you must fight the urge not to read. Managers need to read regularly — professional journals, business publications, annual reports, news magazines, newspapers, anything and everything from MGMA.

Read with an open mind. Read and absorb. Read enough to be sure you have a fix on what's happening in the economy and in your sector of it. Don't just read about the things that relate to the kind of work you do, but look at the discussion of broader trends in your industry. Keep up with your own company. If it's publicly traded, watch its stock. If it's a not-for-profit, check its financial position.

By the way, if you can't find out about your employer, that's a warning sign.

Tim subscribed to all the right journals, but he only looked for articles that would tell him how to do a better job with personnel. He didn't pay attention to other items, so he overlooked published predictions of acquisitions and mergers and the corporatization of health care.

Lynn, Dan, and Linda by contrast not only read, they listened and talked to each other about the things they read.

Linda followed the industry in business publications, paid attention to what crossed her desk, and asked questions. Dan read the *Wall Street Journal, US News & World Report, the Atlanta Constitution*,, as well as everything he could find on MIS. Lynn figured out that Kirkwood was behind the curve in computing and technology. She started reading everything she could find on those subjects and started learning about software related to her work.

Watch the trends

Your options are defined by your knowledge and the assumptions you make based on that knowledge. In addition to reading and following the electronic media, also watch for legislation, regulations, movement by industry, shifts in public opinion, and so forth. In other words, *use* the information you absorb. Analyze it, and ask yourself how it might affect you at work. Always be asking, "What does it mean to me?"

In 1992, Americans expected that health care legislation at the federal level would have a significant impact on health care financing and delivery. In 1994, it became clear that federal government would do nothing. Observers thought that major change would then take place at the state level.

By 1995, it was clear that the real change was emanating from the demands of the business community and from large corporate health care systems, for-profit hospital companies, insurance companies, and integrated systems.

Tim didn't study proposed health care legislation because he just saw that as a government take-over. The idea of purchasing alliances and integrated systems just didn't get his attention. So he was really caught by surprise when the private sector started capitalizing on the fear of government take-over by building bigger and bigger systems.

By contrast Lynn, Dan, and Linda were looking, listening, and checking out what they thought they were seeing and hearing.

Keep your résumé current

For a long time in this country, employees have been pretty safe in assuming that if they showed up for work on time each day, did an OK job, and didn't cause trouble, they could keep their jobs as long as they wanted. Those days are gone for now.

Today, wise employees realize that their companies might go out of business, or that they might be laid off or be asked to transfer to a situation they don't want. Wise employees reflect on this possibility every so often.

We all need to keep our résumés current within a

month or two. We all need to keep a list of the first 10 people we would call if we suddenly needed another job. Keeping your résumé current is a good exercise. It makes you focus on what you're doing. It makes you face the fact that there are no sure things in health care today.

The last time Tim had written a résumé had been 15 years earlier, when he went to work for Kirkwood. He did not plan to change employers so he didn't see the need to update his résumé. His job had changed over time, but he hadn't seen any reason to bring his résumé up to date. Even though he saw résumés constantly in his job at Kirkwood and subsequently with Jones, when he needed to write his, he wasn't sure of what was the preferred method today.

Don't let that happen to you!

Conclusion

Tim was caught totally by surprise and didn't consider his options when his world changed. He considered himself powerless. Reality wasn't as he had perceived it, so he felt lost. He didn't look at how he might stay in Georgia instead of moving to Kansas.

Once he went to Kansas, he still spent all of his time working. He didn't learn anything from the first experience to help him get ready for the next one. There were warning signs all over the place, but Tim didn't see them.

Is Tim an overblown caricature? Yes — but there's a lot of Tim in many of us. Corporate America taught many of us to be tunnel-visioned workaholics.

We all need to spend some time thinking about our options. We need to remind ourselves at regular intervals that things can change. We need to think about how much income we need, what we're willing to put up with, where we're willing to go, and how much lifestyle change is acceptable.

Watching for warning signs and thinking about how to take care of yourself are essential to your well-being. The signs you see may not mean that your company, your practice, or your hospital is being acquired or sold, but they *might* mean exactly that. Be on the lookout for warning signs, and pay close attention to the ones you see.

CHAPTER 6

Build your credibility

The foundations of credibility, as we intend to use the term, are simple: believability, predictability, and honesty.

There is another important factor in the discussion of credibility: perception. *Your* opinion is not what determines your credibility — what matters is how others perceive you. Your creditability is based on *their* perception.

We will make the assumption that our readers are good people trying hard to do a good job in a crazy world not of their making. We assume that you are honest and reliable people. Then we will take all bets that not everyone at your work sees you that way.

Our opinion, not to be confused with reality...

Our good friend Ed Hampe, a clinical psychologist, often starts his comments to his clients by saying, "My opinion, not to be confused with reality...." This preamble enables Ed to say what he thinks, but leaves the client free to disagree. We advocate frequent use of Ed's phrase. It will help you recognize that what you think is real may not be reality, and that what you think is real darned sure probably isn't what someone else thinks reality is.

A difference in perception can result over a very small matter. Jonathan came home late one night after his parents were asleep. He closed the door to the master bedroom before he turned on his TV. The next morning his mother thanked him for being so thoughtful and closing the door so that he would not disturb her sleep. Jonathan started to accept the compliment but then felt guilty and said, "I really did it because you and Dad were both snoring so loudly that I couldn't hear the TV." Clearly the mother's perception of the event differed from Jonathan's.

Likewise on the topic of credibility, different people may have differing perceptions. Your own opinion of your credibility is not very relevant. What matters is the perception of others. Here's a short list of people in your organization whose perceptions matter.

Your bosses. The perception of people above you determines how you are treated. It determines promotions and raises, and it determines your fate if downsizing occurs. If the people above you perceive that you support the organization and will help it achieve its goals, they will retain you. People above you who do not perceive that may fire you.

Your peers. The perceptions of your peers determine whether or not they cooperate with you. Most people today do not believe a medical group manager can succeed as a "Lone Ranger." You must work with others as a team. If your peers don't believe and trust you as a team player, they will find ways to avoid working with you.

Your employees. People below you who perceive that you have credibility will support you; those who don't, won't. If they think that you will look out for them and give them a fair shake, they will help you. Those who do not perceive that will not help you and they may very well actively try to hurt you. Employees who trust their boss will work more effectively than employees who don't.

How to build credibility

Having said all this, the question now is, how does one build credibility? There are five components:

- Do your job;
- Tell the truth;
- Give and keep your word;
- Build and maintain relationships; and
- Help others succeed, recognize their accomplishments, and go to bat for them.

Let's look at these one at a time.

Do your job

The first step in building credibility is to do your job, and do it well. In fact, try to do a great job! If you don't at least do a good job, you will not have credibility. It's this simple — be sure that you know what your job is, do it, do it right and do it on time.

Smart medical practice managers remember to do their jobs. They keep their clinic or their department running on a day-to-day basis. No matter what the chaos of the times, they "keep the trains running," and they manage to get the patient, the medical record and the physician in the same place at the same time. They don't let payroll or billing get fouled up. All mistakes can be serious, but those dealing with someone else's money are high on the list.

Doing your job right is really important. You must pay attention to the basics. We've all lived through the experience of turning in our "best work" only to have the boss, or worse yet, the boss's secretary, find a silly mistake. Ask someone else to proof-read everything you write before you turn it in. Smart managers don't hesitate to ask for help. Make sure there are no misspelled words and make sure that the numbers add up.

You all know war stories about managers who failed to check their work and lost credibility as a result. Here are a few from our experience.

- A personnel supervisor who didn't double check the time sheets and let a silly mistake cost an employee enough on her check that she couldn't pay the utility bill;

- The accountant who gave her boss the wrong year's data for his 7:00 a.m. budget meeting with his boss;

- The CEO who didn't take action on a reported case of sexual harassment;

- The assistant who left a highly confidential document on the copy machine; and

- The Medical Director who overlooked the lack of documentation in a medical record.

Clearly mistakes come in all shapes and sizes; these are but a few samples. Smart managers know that no matter how hard they try, they will make mistakes. They also learn from their mistakes. They know that bosses will question the credibility of an employee who repeats the same mistake too many times.

We don't think that an occasional foul-up scuttles you or causes you to be labeled incompetent. Doing a poor job in one instance labels you as human. Your goal is not to achieve perfection — that's not a realistic business goal. Your goal is to reduce the number and severity of mistakes, and when they occur to accept responsibility and learn from them.

Again, perception is important. It's not enough to do your job, you must be sure that the perception on the part of higher-ups is that you *are* doing it. In today's fast-paced climate, how you are perceived is increasingly based on brief, direct contact with the boss, and on your written products. Frequently your work is reviewed by the boss or someone in the boss's office when you aren't present to explain what you meant. Actual time spent with the boss is becoming more and more limited as people increasingly are tied up in meetings and communicate with cellular phones, E-mail, voice-mail, and fax machines.

Tell the truth

The second component of building credibility is telling the truth. People want to know if what you are saying is true. Some people are more suspicious than others, but everyone has some degree of skepticism about what they hear. It's unpleasant to be treated with skepticism when you are telling the truth. However, it is important to understand that the other person's background may be different from yours; he or she may perceive things very differently.

When you speak or write, the message must be the truth as you know it. In telling the truth it's also important to think about *how* you say or write it. Usually you do not want to slap someone in the face with the truth as if it were a challenge to a duel.

A consultant we know once told a group of internists what they needed to hear. Before he answered their questions he warned them, "If you don't want the truth, don't ask me." He did it deliberately, fully willing to put up with their animosity. This is harder for managers to do than it is for consultants. After all, the consultant does the work and goes away; managers have to stay behind and clean up the mess. Still, there are times when managers have to lay it out bluntly and say that a full disclosure of the facts will be unpleasant.

An employee caught in a lie may be kept around for awhile, but will have lost credibility, perhaps for good. Telling a lie does serious and perhaps permanent damage to one's credibility — it sticks around for a long time. It will take anyone who knows about the lie (and everyone will) a long time to get over it.

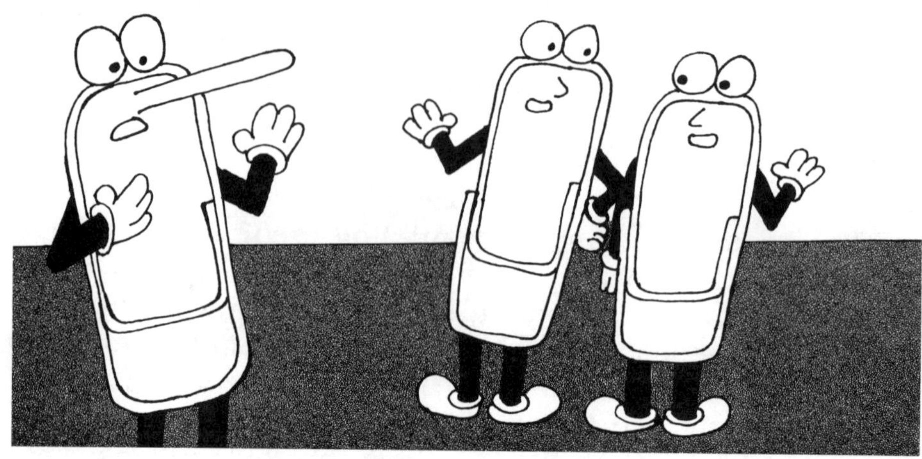

Not telling the truth doesn't just mean telling lies. It also includes withholding information or not being candid. If bosses change the game plan without telling their employees, they are not telling the truth by our definition. They owe it to their staff to keep them informed. And what's true for bosses is equally true for employees. If employees perceive any important change in circumstances within the organization, they have the obligation to report it to management.

Here's an example of someone being less than candid. A clinic administrator had asked for a day off to deal with some personal business. The night before this scheduled day off, he was called at home and asked to come in the next day to meet with his Medical Director and an administrator from MegaHealth on a specific issue related to the sale of his group's practice to MegaHealth. Clearly this was an extremely important meeting so the administrator agreed to come in. When he got to the office the next morning, the Medical Director informed him that the meeting wouldn't be held with the person from MegaHealth, but "I wanted to see you anyway."

The Medical Director proceeded to discuss two or three items that could have easily waited a day, or for that matter a week! The administrator wanted to say, "Next time tell me the truth and let me make the decision whether to give up my time or not. Don't manipulate me." The administrator didn't feel secure enough to say it...but he remembered the event forever.

Over time you develop a reputation for being either truthful or not. If you are thought to be truthful, you are in the game. If the perception is one of not being truthful, the game is over. Of course being truthful alone is not enough. As a manager, if an employee comes to you and says, "I really fouled up on this thing you gave me to do," you may be upset, but the employee will not have lost credibility. But if it happens 10 times in a row, you will probably say, "Well this is an honest guy, but he can't do the job!"

The point: While truthfulness is critical, it cannot stand on its own.

Give your word and keep it

If you do your job and tell the truth, and if people perceive that you do both, you're in good shape. Step three is to give your word, and keep it. We'll illustrate this one with our obligatory war (real war) story — or at least with the movie version of the story.

In the movie "Patton," General Eisenhower's Chief of Staff asks all the commanders if anyone can reach Bastion to relieve the 101st Airborne. General Patton (played by George C. Scott) says, "I can be there in three days." The reaction is at first derision, but as he explains his plan, they all agree to let him try. Their decision to accept his plan was in large part based on the lack of other viable options. General Patton had anticipated the need, and had a plan ready before anyone else. He was able to see the big picture and plan accordingly. While his commitment was bold, it was not foolish.

He reached Bastion in time to save the 101st and stopped Germany's last offensive of World War II. In relieving Bastion, Patton redeemed himself for previous problems and accomplished something that will inspire military people for centuries.

OK, so General Patton gave his word and kept it; he delivered. But isn't this an overblown example that has no relevance to any of us today? Could be, but we know a lot of medical group managers who are being asked to do the impossible today. Some will give their word inappropriately. General Patton had done a very objective analysis of the situation, and gave his word with a high degree of confidence that he could keep it. Many managers today are giving their word even though they know in their hearts that they can't live up to it.

Certainly most of the times when you give your word, the situation doesn't appear to be a life and death matter. However, you might consider it in that context. Word not kept can "kill you" in the work world.

We all know people who will give their word lightly but not keep it. They over-promise and under-deliver. They always have an excuse, but the bottom line is they commit to something that they should not.

Some examples:

- The Administrator of Apex Clinic who gave his word to a large employer that pre-employment physicals would be performed at times convenient to the company — only to find out that the doctors were unable or unwilling to change their schedule;

- The MegaHealth physician known for his temper who promised in a meeting with the employees that his tantrums "will never happen again"; and

- The Administrator at Coyote Healthcare who agreed to an unrealistic deadline for a merger of three separate personnel systems and added that it would be done "without any disruption to patient care."

The higher in the organization you are located, the more serious the consequences for not keeping your word. This is in part because the higher you are, the more people for whom, and to whom, you are responsible. It's also because the higher up you are, the more people there are to watch you. And finally there are always some people in any organization who, with glee, will attempt to do in the higher-ups.

Be sure when you give your word that you have control over all the factors necessary for success. Otherwise give it conditioned on the other things being available. For example, in response to a request to catch up billing say, "I can do it in (blank) days, provided you approve overtime for *x* number of people and/or let me pull in (blank) temps for (blank) days."

Keeping your word also plays a part in confidentiality situations. You've all had the experience of someone coming to you and saying, "Can I talk to you in confidence?" Don't fall into this trap. First, ask the question, "Have you told anyone else?" If the answer is yes, point out that it really isn't confidential any more. Then be sure to say, "I don't know whether I can keep it confidential or not; that will depend on what it is." In this way you can avoid getting caught in a bind between keeping your commitment to silence and doing your duty to the organization.

Build and maintain relationships

It is possible to do your job, tell the truth, and keep your word, but still not have credibility with others. This happens if you have no relationships with others. (Another saying from Ed Hampe: "There must first *be* a relationship before it can be strained.") If relationships don't exist, they must be built. If they exist, they must be maintained. And most of all, they have to be understood.

"Functionalize" relationships.

Relationships are among the major tools that managers use to do their jobs. Just as a carpenter or a mechanic needs a wide variety of tools, a medical group manager needs a variety of relationships. Managers need to be sure that their tool pouch is loaded with a number of functional relationships before they start out to manage an organization or a unit.

What is a functional relationship? It is, for example, the kind of relationship you have with the cashier at the gas station, or the attendant at the subway token booth. The two of you need to work together to accomplish the things you both want to get done.

A functional relationship is not (necessarily) a personal relationship or a friendly relationship or a social relationship. At their heart, functional relationships don't *have* a heart. They exist purely for practical reasons. You can describe functional relationships with words like "civil," "neutral," "transactional," even "mechanical," and you won't hurt their feelings, because they don't have feelings.

For example, physicians who are in the same "call group," can be completely comfortable with the arrangement, even though on a personal level they are not particularly fond of one another. This is possible because they trust each other's professional competence, and because they have built functional relationships.

Of course, human beings are not machines. Most people want to relate to others as people, not as part of some kind of "functional unit." But at work, these wonderful human tendencies must often take a back seat to the simple concept of getting the work done. Seeing to this is one of the constant chores of management.

This is a topic that is broad and deep. Let's look at some of the elements that can produce successful relationships at work. We'll begin with a tip from a physician.

Clarify the relationship.

Dr. Mary Barry is a practicing internist who learned a handy technique when she was a resident in Atlanta. She now passes this technique along to the residents she teaches, and in particular to any female residents who, like Dr. Barry herself, are of average height.

Back in her residency, she noticed that whenever she would lead a gaggle of medical students into patients' hospital rooms on rounds, the patients would invariably scan the group and then fix their vision on the tallest male, obviously expecting that person to be "the doctor." Eventually Dr. Barry discovered the value of walking directly up to the bed with her hand out and her eyes making contact with the patient, while saying in a clear, polite, and unmistakably authoritative voice: "Hello, I'm Dr. Barry... and I am in charge."

What a remarkably easy way to clarify a relationship! We recommend this direct approach in all settings as a way to save time and energy, and to avoid misunderstandings and hurt feedings.

There is a similar trick that works well when you are conducting a meeting. Start the meeting by saying, "Here's our objective, here's our time limit, and here's your role. These rules only cover this meeting." That way you have defined the way the participants will relate, based on the project at hand. Savvy managers give their people all the information they need in language they can understand.

Another aid to clarifying relationships is feedback. Give feedback in the language and style that people demonstrate they use. Your own objectivity is important, and can be obtained by mentally standing back and viewing the situation as if you were watching a play.

Mentally try to put yourself on the other person's side. Avoid making judgments until all the facts are in. Instead of attacking someone who has apparently fouled something up, say, "I don't know if there is anything wrong or not. Here is what I saw and heard...." Then give a simple explanation of what you think the situation is.

Practice feedback listening. Play back to others what they said, or more specifically, your perception of what they said. Note, though, that some people are open and want honest feedback; others are not and do not. Giving honest feedback to someone who is guarded and defensive may earn you a lifetime enemy.

Another good piece of advice about feedback is to "Watch out for blind spots." We all have blind spots, and by definition it is hard for us to see things in our blind spots. Often we don't even know where they are unless someone points them out. Train your staff to help you identify your blind spots. Your enemies will show you your blind spots as they eat your lunch, so you are much better off when people who feel a kinship with you show you your blindspots first.

Clarify expectations.

We have now arrived at one of the truly central concepts related to developing successful relationships at work: clarifying expectations. Some people bring unrealistic expectations to a functional relationship. They come to work expecting warm, fuzzy, feel-good communication, and they are shocked that bosses and co-workers want a functional relationship.

To avoid that kind of shock (and other problems, too), the first step is to focus on expectations. As a manager, ask yourself, "What is the goal or expected outcome of the relationship? What are people willing to do, here and now, for the organization? What do they (and you) expect of the relationship?" These are basic questions that you must ask constantly throughout your day and your career.

This story illustrates the point. The Chief Operating Officer for a fast-growing managed care company was walking through the office one afternoon when she ran into Mike, the Provider Relations manager. The COO said, "Mike, you're doing a really nice job keeping our providers happy. Things couldn't be going better. There will be a nice surprise in your paycheck tomorrow."

Mike was thrilled at first just to be recognized, but as the day passed, he focused more and more on his "raise." By the time he got his check the next afternoon he was expecting thousands. He got a $100 per month raise. A very nice gesture, except it did not come close to his expectations, which were inflated because of the boss's remark. The COO gave a sincere compliment to Mike, but then should have said specifically "I've authorized a $100 increase in your pay, just to let you know we've noticed the good results you're getting."

A slight twist on clarifying expectations: What do you do when you hear people saying, "We don't believe management will do anything to solve the problems?"

This is not just a statement about expectations; it is also an indictment of management. As a manager, you want to help your staff change this expectation, if it is inaccurate; or change the organization, if their perception is accurate.

There *are* organizations that won't do anything. We read about sexual harassment and physical abuse being ignored. We read that workers say top management "just doesn't get it." If top management is viewed this way by the troops, it will be hard to motivate people to put out extra effort or to do their jobs to the peak of their abilities. *Your* credibility will suffer.

Don't go looking for love in all the wrong places.

Most managers secretly wish employees would leave their personal and family problems at home, along with their social and political agendas, and most of all their unfulfilled romantic needs. That'll be the day. As we said before, people are not machines, and it is unrealistic for managers to hope that employees will behave like robots.

The toughest kind of relationship is the office romance. The traditional wisdom on this subject says that management should discourage romantic involvements among coworkers. The authors support that view. Remember, the topic of this chapter is credibility. It is nearly impossible for a manager to maintain credibility when the manager is playing matchmaker or when the manager is involved in a strong personal relationship with someone at work. In those cases, employees and even bosses will have good reason to question the manager's objectivity.

The workplace is not a proper place for people to look for unqualified love, but for whatever reasons, people do just that. This fascinating topic is beyond the scope of this book. But management problems certainly crop up in this area, and the problems will not go away just because managers wish they would. Let's consider some fundamental truths that managers should understand and abide by.

First, the line between seeking approval and seeking affection can be treacherously thin. Everyone in the work force wants to be recognized for their accomplishments, and good managers will respond to that need by providing the support and recognition and attention that employees want and deserve. And that is where it must end. For managers it is absolutely critical to keep one's personal life and professional life separate and distinct. Of course, if "liking someone too much" can be a problem for some people, so can the opposite condition. Second, in the workplace, people don't have to like each other to have a perfectly good functional relationship. Certainly it is natural for people to want to be liked, and to feel more comfortable when they work around people they are fond of. But that can't happen all the time. Managers who can help people understand how to make functional relationships work can have an enormous and positive effect on morale and efficiency.

Having fun and getting to know people at work can be fine, but it must be secondary to the formation of a functional relationship. As in most things, these tough issues require judgment and balance. Caring about the employees, showing you care, wanting the best for them, telling them you are proud of them...these are examples of positive, appropriate, and re-affirming actions and passions. These are to be encouraged among managers. But becoming too involved in the personal affairs, the financial dealings, or the emotional lives of employees is a great danger, and must be avoided.

Help others succeed, recognize their accomplishments, and go to bat for them

This is the fifth component of building credibility. Some will say that this topic is really part of building and maintaining relationships. Clearly that could be the case. We chose to make it a separate section because we think it deserves that level of attention.

Managers need to be candid when they look in the mirror and ask themselves, "How do I treat employees?" Your real power comes from people above and below you. True, power is given to managers when they are appointed to their positions. However, that power can be fleeting and elusive if the manager fails to understand and work appropriately with people at all levels. Ultimately, success does not come because you have power over people, but because you empower people, give them credit and stand up for them.

If people believe that you want them to succeed, they will work harder for you and for the organization. You show it daily by positive feedback, by pointing out to your boss that someone below you contributed to something that the boss likes, by nominating them for awards, by making sure that they get raises and upgrades as appropriate...and by standing up to the boss.

There comes a time in every manager's career when you have to take on the boss over something related to one of your employees. Our only caution is, in the words of Davy Crockett, "Be sure you're right and go ahead."

If you're not right, watch out. We've all had the experience of standing up for an employee only to have the boss prove to us that we were wrong.

Here's a two-part example of what happened when a manager went to bat for an employee and won with both the boss and the employee.

I'm not fussing at you. I'm just fussing.

"I wasn't fussing at her, I was fussing in general," Dr. Godley told his administrator Ms. Smart when she asked him what he had said to Missy, the appointments and registration supervisor.

Ms. Smart had worked for Dr. Godley long enough to know when she could challenge him and how to do it. This was one of those times, so she looked him square in the eye and said, "You feel better because you got it off your chest, but now you've messed up the organization for a week!"

She was subtly reminding him that he had to take responsibility for his actions and for the fall-out.

He didn't apologize to me.

"Point well taken," Dr. Godley said to Ms. Smart. "Tell Missy I'm sorry."

Feeling that she had communicated her concern to Dr. Godley and that he understood the situation, she thought everything would soon be back to normal. But when she told Missy about it, Missy's response was, "Why didn't he apologize to me himself?"

At that point Ms. Smart made a crucial decision. She went back to Dr. Godley and told him, "I would like you to talk to Missy yourself. She's good at the job. Appointments and registration get done, patients and physicians rarely wait, and we can't afford to lose her." After some storming about, shouting things like, "I won't be blackmailed..." and "Who does she think she is?..." Dr. Godley agreed to call Missy and apologize.

Not every medical group manager could, or should, do this. But if you know your staff and you know your doctors, there are times when you have to take a stand. We also know that managers who have reputations for standing up for their employees are usually well-respected, effective, and credible.

Conclusion

Credibility is based on believability, predictability, and honesty. Most important, your credibility rests on others' perceptions of how you stack up related to those qualities. To build credibility, you must do your job, tell the truth, give and keep your word, build and maintain relationships, and help others succeed.

It's not rocket science, but it is hard work. It takes constant attention. Credibility is hard to gain and easy to lose.

CHAPTER 7

Build your political skills

"Political skills." UGH! We don't want to talk about politics in a book about something as pure and noble as running a medical facility, do we?

Well, actually...yes, we do.

Any word that stems from the term "politics" is a dirty word to many people who are disgusted with the actions or inactions of their government at all levels — federal, state, and local. Likewise many people condemn "office politics," which they see as an effort by someone else to get ahead on something other than merit. They see politics as misusing people and resorting to "dirty tricks."

The authors don't share these negative beliefs about politics and political skills. We define political skills as the ability to shape the behavior of individuals and organizations, to the extent of your persuasive and coercive power. This means interaction with other people to accomplish goals. Without such interactions no one could ever be successful.

Good politics means using good people (political) skills. People (political) skills are essential for successful management. Managers must build their people (political) skills to take care of themselves, to take care of their organizations, and to have credibility within their organizations.

Using political skill doesn't mean pulling the wool over someone's eyes, or thriving at someone else's expense. It means looking for the win/win situation, not the win/lose. Politically smart managers know that if other people feel they lose in encounters with them, they won't cooperate.

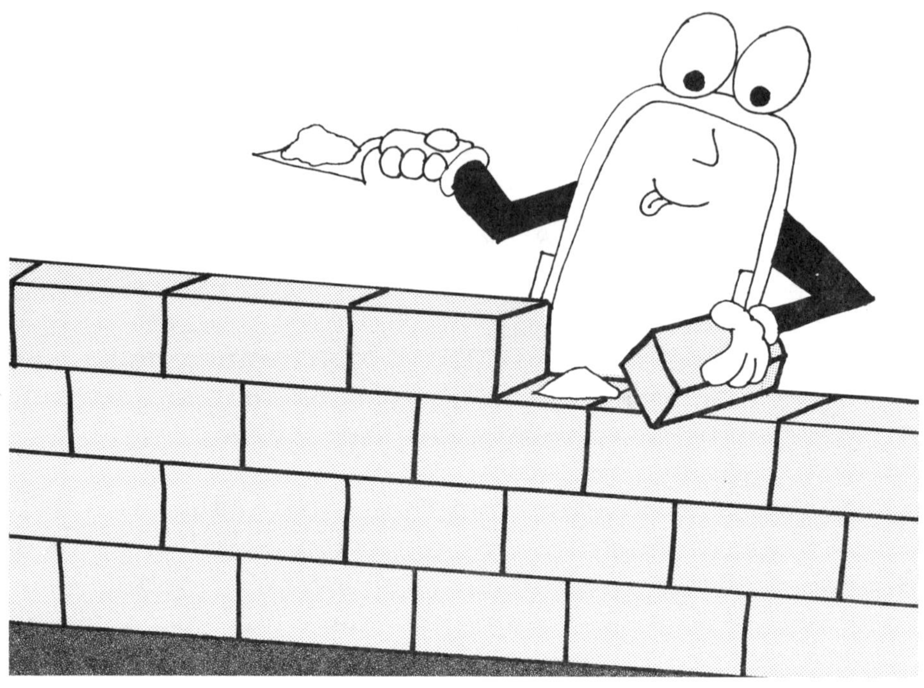

Let's look at how two medical group managers of equal talent but differing political skills handled themselves and their jobs in a changing environment, and at how they each fared in the process. We have to start out telling you about the physicians they worked for, Dr. Godley and Dr. Peacock.

The Short, Smart story

Dr. Godley, like nearly every physician in America, had been reading professional journals and going to meetings and seminars where he was hearing that medical practice was changing. The messages he was getting were, "We're going to managed care; we're going to have less income; we're going to have to worry about keeping people healthy; continuity of care is essential; etc."

In Dr. Godley's world, the only time "change" was defined as "good" was when it was initiated by Dr. Godley. All other change was evil and was to be avoided. Now he was being told he must make changes because of external forces, and that things were going to be very different in his medical practice from the way they had been for the past 20 years.

This did not sound like fun to Dr. Godley.

Dr. Godley was a powerful man who was always in charge. Many people (including Dr. Godley himself!) considered him to be the best family practitioner in town. He had put together a group of seven other family practitioners, a group which was considered by many to be a premiere practice. He had a gratis faculty appointment at the medical school where he lectured students and residents on the merits of physicians controlling their professional lives and maximizing their income in small, single-specialty groups.

Everything had been perfect for Dr. Godley. His world had been to his liking: it was a world largely defined and built by him. Now rather suddenly, somebody else was changing health care. He didn't understand what was happening or why, but he knew sinister forces were at work. He wasn't sure who was behind these changes or what they wanted, but he darned sure didn't like it.

In the past, people describing Dr. Godley's personality might have said "he's sometimes volatile." These days they dropped the "sometimes." His administrator, Ms. Smart, was frequently on the receiving end of his tantrums.

After going through the phases of grief, denial, and anger several times, Dr. Godley finally decided to act. He listened to the experts who told him to "do something" — merge, expand, join a hospital, affiliate, create a physician/hospital organization, etc. In the absence of clear-cut knowledge about what to do, but being a doer, he did something. He got with Dr. Peacock, the head of a five-physician family medicine group in the area, and started talking about merging their practices.

Dr. Peacock was a meticulous person who worried about the appearance of the facility, the attire of the staff, and many other details of medical practice operations. Like Dr. Godley he was concerned about his ability or inability to control his future. Dr. Peacock seldom felt "out of control," but the changing environment was making him irritable.

Dr. Peacock and his administrator, Ms. Short, had worked together for seven years. They understood each other. She made sure that everything, every day, met his exacting standards for cleanliness and orderliness. There was a process for everything, and the process was followed. There was a place for everything, and everything was in its place.

Why me, Lord?

When the intent to merge was announced, life started getting much more stressful for Ms. Smart and Ms. Short, who felt like the rug had been pulled from under them. If they didn't ask the question, "Why me, Lord?" out loud, they certainly thought it!

They were told by their respective physicians something to this effect: "It's up to you to make this merger happen smoothly. If you do, we'll see that you'll come out OK. Um, we'll tell you later who is going to be head of what and where you fit in."

Both were bright, well-educated and experienced administrators. Both were candidates in the American College of Medical Practice Executives. They both tried to stay current in reading the literature of their field. They attended MGMA annual meetings and regional conferences, and were active with their state chapter and the local branch. Both saw themselves on the "cutting edge" in terms of knowing practice management.

As managers of well-respected groups, both Ms. Smart and Ms. Short were viewed by their peers as leaders in their field. Up to this stage in their careers nothing pinpointed which one was a more effective administrator than the other.

Their responses

All the uncertainty over the merger caused stress for everyone involved, but perhaps most of all for these two administrators. They were challenged to work harder than they had ever worked and to get more done than they had ever done before, while keeping their practices running. They had to keep morale up in the face of the pending changes. They had to plan and implement change while living with the uncertainty of where they fit into the picture in the new combined operation. They had to address differences in everything from the specific, such as the different retirement plans, to the intangible, such as the differing cultures.

They responded very differently. Ms. Short saw the situation as an unanticipated problem; Ms. Smart saw it as a welcomed opportunity. Ms. Short focused on tried-and-true processes to solve the "problem." Ms. Smart focused on political skills to respond to the "opportunity." Their differing attitudes had an impact on the outcome for both.

The Short response. Ms. Short went into her office and started working on organizational charts, staffing patterns, ideas for combining departments, etc. She came early, stayed late, and carried bundles of work home every night. She called MGMA for a literature search, and she read journals and books on mergers. She knew that she needed to spend extra hours reading, writing and thinking about the merger if she was to come out on top.

She felt she had to do the extra work in addition to her already heavy work load. It might not come as a surprise that she developed a short fuse and started blowing up frequently. She was not happy with her own behavior all the time, but she felt her staff should understand that she was fighting for them, and she thought they should be tolerant of her outbursts.

The Smart response. Initially, Ms. Smart was also stressed out. She had been given too many new Top Priority tasks to add to the stack of *old* Top Priority tasks. None of the old projects went away, but instead they had to be interwoven with the overriding issue of merging the practices. She couldn't quite figure it all out. She got to the point of wanting to change jobs. She actually thought she might be on the road to a nervous breakdown.

Then she decided to take care of herself by taking a day off.

Like any good overworked manager, she took her work home in her briefcase. When she got up the next day, after a good night of sleep, she ate a leisurely breakfast and read the paper. Later as she walked through her study and saw the briefcase, a light came on for her and everything became clear. Within a short time she had listed on one page the really major tasks that needed to be done in the next six months on the merger project. How major is "really major?" Here is an example: "Keep the medical practice running smoothly" was one single item on her list.

She then started going through each piece of paper in her briefcase and checked it against her list. If it didn't fit, she set it aside. After two hours she had a matrix with every task and sub-task that needed to be done to achieve the goals of the original list. She placed items that didn't fit in a separate file, to be addressed later.

She took the matrix to the next supervisory staff meeting two days later. She gave everyone a copy and reviewed it at some length. She then passed around an original and asked people to initial the things for which they felt responsible.

After the matrix circled the table, it came back to her with two or more sets of initials by some items, and no initials next to others. She asked people to look at it again and see who would take responsibility for items that no one had initialed the first time. She also asked them to review the items where two or more had been initialed to determine who was willing to swap what.

Through this process she got her staff to accept this work plan as being their own work plan for the next six months. After two more trips around the table, the list was complete, with one person responsible for each item on the matrix. They then spent the next hour working on the time frame.

I'm here to help you

As frequently happens with physicians, Dr. Peacock and Dr. Godley changed signals in the middle of the merger. They became convinced that they needed a consultant to act as a facilitator.

Neither Ms. Smart nor Ms. Short felt that the consultant was needed at this point. They had worked out many issues between them. They would have admitted that some consultation was needed, but they resented the project being turned over to an outsider in mid-stream.

Ms. Smart took a deep breath, counted to 10 and said to herself, "OK, it's Dr. Godley's money, and if he wants to spend it on an unnecessary consultant to make him feel better, fine." She then approached the consultant with an attitude of cooperation, and tried hard to communicate effectively. She worked late a few nights to get the consultant everything he asked for, and to identify other things that she thought he would need.

Ms. Short's approach was the opposite. She resented the consultant and let him know it non-verbally. Working with her was difficult for the consultant. Ms. Short was always busy, even harried. The consultant didn't get anything from her without asking for it several times, and then it was seldom what he wanted or needed.

The outcome

It should not come as a surprise what the outcome was. Ms. Smart communicated; Ms. Short isolated herself. Ms. Smart asked her staff to help her and they responded. Ms. Short blew up at her staff if they interrupted her "very important work."

Although there were definitely some rough spots, Ms. Smart kept Dr. Godley's medical practice on the right track while working toward the merger. Morale may have dipped a little, but it remained at a reasonable level. Patients were seen, bills were sent, and revenue continued.

Dr. Peacock's practice had a different experience. The employees started bickering. Appointments got fouled up. Patients came at the "wrong time" or didn't come at all. Worst of all, two weeks worth of billing got lost!

When the consultant finished he recommended (surprise!) that Ms. Smart become the administrator of the combined operation and that Ms. Short not be retained. He didn't feel that Ms. Short had the right attitude, skills or ability to be productive in the number two position. However, true to his word, Dr. Peacock demanded that a slot be found for her. She was offered the position of assistant administrator, but with hurt feelings turned it down.

It's all politics

Was Ms. Smart smarter than Ms. Short? On an I.Q. test, probably not. Did she have more street smarts? Unquestionably.

The real difference in the two was political skill. Ms. Short was not aware of the need for political skills, she only thought in terms of work skills. Ms. Smart would not use the term political skills, instead she would talk about "working with people" and about "being tuned in to what's happening," and so forth. However, she was political in the best sense of the word. What were the specific political skills that Ms. Smart used? Here is a list.

Be conscious of your power base.

If you don't take care of your own power base, you can't take care of yourself or your organization. It is absolutely essential to know and understand the base of your power. You must assess how power is used and shared in your organization and you must assure your power base through relationships.

Ms. Smart recognized quickly that the arrival of the consultant caused a shift of some power away from her and Ms. Short, at least temporarily. Ms. Short saw the consultant as an annoyance, and failed to recognize or respect his power. Nor did she realize that her own power had been diminished.

Know your boundaries.

Assigned power won't cover up incompetence very long. To succeed you must find your niche, know your limits, negotiate an understanding with your superiors about what *is* your job and what *is not*. (The "*is not*" is just as important as the "*is*.") Otherwise managers end up losing credibility or being blamed for something over which they have no control.

It is important to remember that others may not know what your boundaries are. A simple conversation can clear up a misunderstanding. It's very likely that in almost any human interaction, the other person will not see it the way you see it. It becomes imperative that you communicate to clarify — particularly in a time of high stress.

Ms. Short failed to realize that boundaries can and do shift, particularly when there is significant change in the environment.

Be competent.

This is simple, solid advice: do your job well. If you don't, political skill will be wasted. Yes, there are always people who can get by on connections, charm, connivance, or something other than merit. And yes, there are competent, deserving managers who don't prosper because of simple bad luck. But under the middle of the bell-shaped curve, the success of most managers depends very heavily on how well they do their jobs. As indicated above, part of "doing your job" is being sure that you and the boss have the same expectation regarding your job. Historically, both Ms. Short and Ms. Smart had exhibited competence. In a changing environment Ms. Smart continued to do so by keeping her clinic running, providing everything the consultant wanted, and keeping her staff informed. Her outlook and her approach made her problems seem smaller, more manageable. Although Ms. Short had historically displayed a high degree of competence in a stable situation, she did not display competence in a changing and stressful environment. Certainly she did some things well during this period, but nothing ran as well as it had in the past and no one was happy with her attitude or the outcome.

Listen.

When significant change happens, get all the information you can and make informed decisions. Listen without preconceived notions. What is going on in *your* head may not be what is going on in someone else's.

Ms. Smart made it a habit to say frequently, "Let me tell you my understanding of this situation, and then please tell me yours." A good technique.

Good managers listen more than they talk. They listen to everyone — bosses, patients, employees, other managers, friends, family, and neighbors. They listen for hints about problems (a.k.a. opportunities), anger, hurt feelings, and unusual comments or unusual silences. One day while strolling through the clinic, Ms. Smart ran into a usually happy employee who appeared to be in a bad mood. Turns out that the employee's paycheck had been short one day's pay because of a processing error, and as a result the rent check bounced. Embarrassed, the employee wasn't going to mention it, but all it took was Ms. Smart saying, "You doin' OK?" for the floodgates to burst open.

In no time at all Ms. Smart had the payroll records fixed, and had a check for the adjustment on its way to the bank, and (because most banks love most medical organizations), she even got the bank to waive the normal $20 penalty — all because Ms. Smart did a bit of routine observation and analysis.

By contrast, one day Ms. Short walked by her billing office, where the same four staffers had worked together in cramped quarters for more than two years, and heard nothing — only cold silence!

So what? Silence is what you want to hear from your billing staff, isn't it? That depends.

If Ms. Short had been alert, she would have realized this was the first time she had ever heard complete silence in that area. In fact, she had in the past wondered how they could do a good job of billing with the constant chatter that seemed to go on.

On this particular day she was too preoccupied to notice the difference. Since she didn't hear the silence as something to investigate, she did nothing. It was weeks later before she learned about the interpersonal issues that had torn her billing office apart and caused two weeks' worth of billing to get lost!

Move, both physically and psychologically.

On most days, if you've been in your office for more than two hours at a time "working behind closed doors," you're not doing your job. You need to be seen by your employees, and they need to feel that you are accessible. Having an open-door policy will allow people to feel free to communicate with you.

As noted before, Ms. Short worked hard in the isolation of her office. She had always done this to an extent, but she became almost totally unavailable during this period. Her staff knew not to interrupt her and break her concentration. Trusting no one to help her, she tried to do it all.

By contrast, it was rare for Ms. Smart to let more than two or three hours pass without a swing through the office. She moved around talking, listening, and observing.

Take action when necessary.

When you hear something that is disturbing to you, take the time to think through what you've heard. Determine what the best course of action would be, if any, and then take it. The fact that you take action may be more important to your staff than the specific action you take.

Ms. Smart walked out into her clinic at 2:30 one afternoon and ran into Paulette, one of the medical assistants. She greeted her with, "How are you, Paulette?" The reply came so quickly that it surprised both Ms. Smart and Paulette. Paulette blurted out, "I'd be a lot better if I'd had lunch!"

Ms. Smart went directly to Paulette's supervisor, Mary, and asked why Paulette had missed lunch. Mary didn't know. In fact, Mary had been at her desk for four straight hours and didn't know that Paulette had missed lunch.

Ms. Smart lectured Mary on the wage and hour labor laws that mandate lunch breaks, and she spoke to her pointedly about allowing Paulette in particular to miss lunch, because Paulette has diabetes. Mary moved quickly to check out the schedules and to take appropriate corrective action.

One more thing: The next day Ms. Smart apologized to Mary for being a bit harsh with her. She thanked Mary for addressing the situation and for helping take care of employees and follow regulations. In the end both Paulette and Mary felt good about Ms. Smart and knew that she cared about them, about their work, and about the organization they all were part of.

In contrast, since Ms. Short was cloistered in her office, often she did not know when action was needed, much less be available to take it.

Be loyal.

Organizational loyalty isn't what it used to be, but that doesn't mean it is not important at all. Among other things, loyalty means being faithful and keeping your word. We feel strongly about it. Here are a couple of blunt truths:

- If you cannot be loyal to your organization and your boss, you need to find other employment; and

- If you cannot be loyal to the people who work under you, they will not be loyal to you.

Loyalty is built over time. Managers have to prove themselves to bosses, peers, and employees. Loyalty starts with giving credit to your employees. Politically smart managers share power, and in particular they share recognition with the people who work for them. A manager gains employees' respect by sharing recognition and praise and by taking responsibility for mistakes.

Politically skilled managers seldom let themselves become impressed with how important they are. Instead they focus on how well their organization runs, and they give credit to everyone else for success. Managers without political skill frequently "put someone in their place" by letting them know who is in charge.

Ms. Smart believed in working with people's strengths, and she believed in empowering her employees. She always went out of her way to make sure the doctors knew when any of the staff did something special. She gave positive feedback constantly, and she corrected people in a positive way.

Again by contrast, as the stress of the merger wore on, Ms. Short began to complain to the physicians about the staff. She was increasingly dissatisfied with the amount or quality of work.

Sometimes "just do it."

There are times to roll up your sleeves, get down and dirty, and do some ordinary work. Dan managed a 10-physician specialty practice which had been in the same location for seven years. During that time a lot of "stuff" had accumulated and had been crammed into storage space. (A truism: No medical practice ever has enough office or storage space.) The need for storage had consumed two exam rooms, a physician's office, and all the closets.

One day Dan decided, "We're gonna clean house." He rented warehouse space, had a dumpster delivered for the trash, and rented a truck to haul the non-junk to a warehouse.

In his next staff meeting he announced that he was going to start house-cleaning the following Saturday morning and would appreciate some help. Five employees showed up on Saturday and sweated through six hours of dirty, grimy work with him. Most of them had never seen

Dan in anything but a suit, and were amazed that he would get down in the trenches and work with them. He gained a lot of respect and loyalty from those five and others on the staff as the word spread.

Don't play it too safe.

Constant communication (especially asking and listening) will alert you when something needs fixing and when it doesn't. At some point, when something needs fixing, you must run the risk of saying so. Playing it safe is a sure way *out* of a job in some circumstances. If bad things happen because a manager was afraid to rock the boat a little, the ship may sink with the manager in it.

Be flexible.

When things start changing, managers must be ready to change. The development of multiple options is essential. Ms. Short immediately took the position, "I know the outcome I want," and closed off other possibilities. She had a single goal — to be in charge of the new combined entity. She wasn't interested in other possibilities.

Ms. Smart kept her options open. Early on she recognized that she might not be the administrator of the new combined operation. She reasoned that since it was a bigger unit, she might have as much money and status in a second-level position as she currently had as the manager in her current position. She also recognized that if this merger was successful, the organization might continue to merge with other entities and one department eventually might be bigger than her whole medical practice was right now.

Now let's explore why political skills are important regardless of the setting.

If only...!

Ms. Short did not go quietly; she alternated between tantrums and paranoia. She accused everyone of conspiring against her. She toyed with a wrongful-discharge lawsuit, but could not find a competent attorney who would take her case without money up front. When she was feeling particularly sorry for herself, she would say something like, "If I'd been working for Dr. Godley and Ms. Smart for Dr. Peacock, this would have turned out differently!"

This is an intriguing theory but one that seldom holds up under scrutiny. In fact, this is a variation of the old "If I could just get a whole new staff..." complaint.

Our advice is look in the mirror — where you will see everything you need to manage (and everything that you can control) to achieve success. If you want to change bosses or change your boss's behavior, first look at yourself. Make sure you aren't part of the problem. Think about what you may need to change to make things work better.

Bosses are like other people — complex mixes of good and bad traits. Both Dr. Godley and Dr. Peacock were highly competent and respected physicians with strong negative and positive personality traits. Either could have been a problem on certain days or in certain situations for any manager. Surprised? Don't be: they were both human. Given the inevitable hierarchy in a medical organizations, managers usually have to accommodate physicians more than physicians have to accommodate managers. Dr. Godley was prone to blow up. Ms. Smart had frequently bit her tongue when that happened. But after it was over she would go to his office and say, "Let's talk." She had learned that they could talk through whatever was bothering him, and that he would back her up when necessary.

The point: She probably would have figured out how to work with Dr. Peacock just as well. Dr. Peacock was not a volatile employer, but, instead, avoided conflict at all costs. He waited to see who was right and then agreed with them. It fell to Ms. Short to confront any and everybody. All complaints landed on her desk. She chewed out employees and fought with other medical practices and with vendors. In stable circumstances Ms. Short was an effective manager. She was technically competent. Before merger talks started, the Peacock Clinic ran well and staff did their jobs. There was a sense of continuity — doing the same thing this year as last year. Political skill was not critical in that environment.

When everything started changing, then political skill became very important. A technically competent person who has not cultivated good political skills cannot develop them overnight. Ms. Short's lack of political skill killed her chances to make the transition to the new organization.

The point again: Working with Dr. Godley would have been unpleasant and unproductive for Ms. Short in those same circumstances, just as it was at Dr. Peacock's clinic.

Conclusion

Ms. Smart appeared to be politically astute, always doing the right thing. Ms. Short appeared to be totally inept and lacking in political skill. It seemed these were two people at complete opposite ends of the spectrum. In reality, all of us have both Smart and Short behavior in us on any given day. Most of us, most days, are not at either extreme, but are somewhere in between. Clearly, the daily goal for managers should be to have *smart* rather than *short* responses.

Even if you employ all of your political skills and do everything right, things may not work out the way you want. Political skills do not assure the outcome you want. Nothing does. Political skills improve your odds and make you more effective; they assure you a better shot at influencing the outcome. Political skills are the icing on the cake, but the substance (knowledge, education, experience and job skill) must still be underneath.

CHAPTER 8

Build your power

Dorothy wanted to get back to Kansas. The good witch didn't have the power to get Dorothy back to Kansas, but said the Wonderful Wizard of Oz did have that power. So Dorothy and Toto, seeing no choice but to begin where they were, started their journey down the Yellow Brick Road. Along the way they picked up some traveling companions who were also looking for someone with the power to change their lives.

So let's begin with where you are. The work load is increasing. The work force is decreasing. Revenue is shrinking. Your patients demand more attention. Employees line up outside your door to complain. Your superiors cut in at the head of the line. The physicians interrupt your superiors. All the lights on your phone blink: Medicare on line one; Utilization Review on line two; an attorney on line three. The computer crashed, and three employees quit.

You feel overwhelmed, crushed, and adrift, with no power to change your situation. You feel like you've been picked up by a tornado, and you are wondering where it will drop you.

Dorothy found she had the power to go home, the Tin Man discovered his heart, the Lion's courage welled up, and the Scarecrow figured out that he could figure things out. They all found what was needed inside themselves. Their premise was wrong: only a wonderful someone else could give them power. The message in this chapter is clear and simple: *You have power!* We want to tell you that, right now, as you face the flying monkeys and wicked witches on health care's yellow brick road. The power to change your situation is inside you.

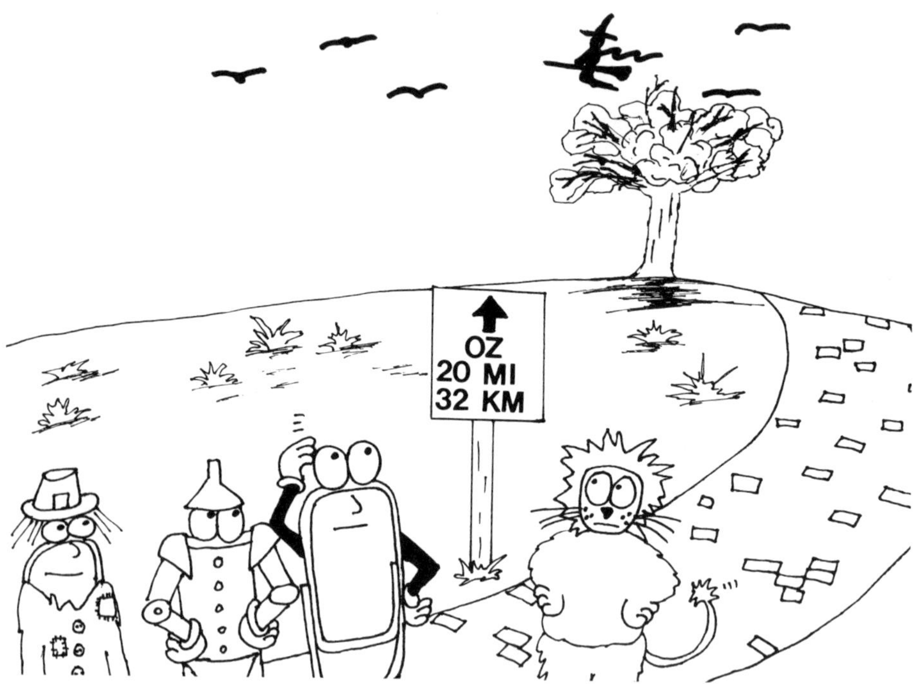

Physicians, administrators, managers, and employees may feel powerless in the storm now raging. That premise is wrong. You have power unless you give it away. This chapter is about identifying your power, retaining it, building it, and using it to take care of yourself and to take care of your organization.

Way down the food chain

Many people feel uncomfortable with the topic of power. They associate power with taking over companies, laying off employees. They see the use of power as disagreeable, even sinister. Their minds link power to such things as scheming, manipulation, and profits at the expense of decency. To them, power means "the law of the jungle," and they feel they are way down on the food chain.

It does not have to be that way. Some managers use power to treat people with respect and to make organizations responsive to human needs. That use of power rejects sinister scheming and manipulation. That approach to power encourages everyone to take intelligent risks to improve themselves and the organization.

The bottom line about power is that nothing in human life ever gets done without people using power. As managers, we *must* use power to achieve anything. *How* we build and use power are the only choices about it.

You have power, unless you give it away. We'll emphasize that point with a true story.

Meet Mr. Sam

"Mr. Sam, can you hear me? Do you know where you are?" Mr. Sam felt like he was encased in a soft-boiled egg, but the insistent voice cut through it. He opened his eyes, looked around, saw the nurse and the oxygen tubes, and said, "Well, from the look of things, I would say I'm in a hospital."

"That's right," said the nurse. "Do you know how you got here?" He replied, "No. Last night I was spray painting my truck. Went to bed with a headache. Today I wake up here." "What night were you working on your truck?" said the nurse. "Monday." "This is Thursday," she said. "Looks like I lost a couple of days," he replied.

To know Mr. Sam is to like him. He is an 84-year-old, center-city resident who gives new meaning to the words "self-directed." Mr. Sam reads Cicero in Latin. He built his own television set in the 1950's, and friends still ask him to repair cars and appliances. He owned a tavern and several other businesses during his working career, while he held down a civil service "day job." He acknowledges with humor that someone else may have to worry with the finishing touches on the basement remodeling job he just started.

Doctor Mannerly (who wasn't) barged in and, interrupting the nurse, stared at Mr. Sam and proclaimed, "You could have a serious problem."

"I was painting my truck and didn't have enough air," Mr. Sam said. "I'm all right now."

Dr. Mannerly continued as though Mr. Sam were a statue. "You were brought in unconscious. You have to get some tests to see what's wrong." "I think I'm OK now," said Mr. Sam: "I think it was just the paint fumes..."

His words were left hanging in the air as the doctor brushed past the nurse on his way out, calling out orders for a battery of tests for "the patient in 3 East 4-B."

Mr. Sam was searching unsuccessfully for his clothes when an orderly came with a gurney and took him to the lab. Mr. Sam said, "I don't want these tests." He got up, carefully reached behind to close the drafty gown, and scooted with back to the wall to the information desk to ask for the loan of a quarter to call his brother. When the desk refused him credit, he walked out the front door, hailed a taxi, and went home. "So you checked out?" a neighbor asked. "No, I didn't check out, I left," Mr. Sam replied.

Mr. Sam may or may not have been right about the paint fumes. Luckily, six months later he had yet to experience any more symptoms. But even if he was not right about the fumes, he was right about something else. He understood that he had power, and that the surest way to lose it is to give it away. He used his power when he exercised his right to leave the hospital, even though it was against medical advice.

Mr. Sam did not have absolute power — nobody does. Like everyone, physical limitations and sometimes the authority of others can limit his power. (As examples, if Mr. Sam were unable to walk, or were younger and in a military hospital, then the story would end differently.) But as long as he reserved for himself the right to act on his own behalf and in his own self-interest, and as long as he did not give that right away, he had power.

In this story, Mr. Sam didn't want any tests. But would

it change the picture if he HAD wanted them, or if he agreed, even skeptically, to have them done? Perhaps. But he was not willing to put his self-interest in the hands of the doctor without a discussion. That would be giving away his power.

Mr. Sam did not give away his power. He thought he had a say in matters of his self-interest. He contemplated risk and chose the risks he would take. He taught the first lesson of power. If you don't make your own choices, someone else might make them for you — and that person might not be acting on your behalf and in your self-interest.

As a case example, look no further than your local version of MegaHealth, a company that buys medical practices and hospitals. Ask yourself if large organizations in a feeding frenzy of acquisitions seem to have a record of watching out for the self-interest of the physicians and the employees when they acquire organizations.

How power works

Power is like good comedy, and Johnny Carson is one of the masters. He often evoked anticipatory giggles from the Tonight Show audience as he set up a joke. Somctimes, he evoked groans in fleshing out the details and the joke fell flat. He would then say, "Hey, if you buy the premise, you buy the bit." With that statement he managed to convey the idea that, once the audience started down the comedic road with him, they had an obligation to complete the journey and laugh at the punch line — even if it wasn't funny.

Surprisingly, power operates in much the same way in the workplace. It has a premise, leading to the details and obligations. Buy the premise, and the details make sense. Then, what you are obligated to do flows logically and must be accepted.

That's what is going on when, for example, you are told that the data from the old software system cannot be converted and loaded into the new system. If you buy that as the only true premise, then you and your staff must work nights and weekends re-keying and verifying the data. The premise, details, and obligations make painful, weary sense, so everyone rolls up their sleeves and puts in the hours.

Power is determined by the premise you buy; your understanding and misunderstanding of the details; and the statements of the resulting obligations. As we shall see later, these three factors are also leverage points for building your power.

When Dorothy bought the premise that only the Wizard of Oz had the power to get her home, she had no choice but to start down the Yellow Brick Road.

Don't give your power away

The title of this chapter is "Build Your Power." As we said in the beginning, the first step in building your power is to be sure you don't give away the power you already have. Many people do not think of themselves as having power, so they are not aware of how they give it away.

Sure enough, if the registration staff thinks they don't have the power to decrease the waiting time for patients and providers, they can't do it. They won't even look for ways to do it, and they give their power to make changes to someone else. Acting powerless robs them of opportunities, options, and sources of job satisfaction.

Here are more examples of ways we dilute or diminish our power:

Not speaking up gives your power away.

Jenny worked for months around a problem her boss created in by assigning her the data-collection task for a research project — on top of her regular Medical Records duties. As a result, Jenny was constantly behind. Finally, the boss demanded better performance. Jenny said, "If you will just let me change the way you asked me to collect and record the data, I can keep up with the work." "Is that the problem? Why didn't you tell me?" demanded the boss. "I knew it would be a problem when you gave me the assignment," said Jenny."

The boss has the right to expect employees to use their power by indicating problems and outlining alternatives. We also think that doing so is one critical way to take care of yourself and your organization. Jenny did neither.

Telling people they are wrong gives power away. According to the late Jim Croce, "You don't pull the mask off the old Lone Ranger...." When you want to get the bosses' attention, you get it another way. In an organization under the control of others, you have only the power they want you to have. You can increase that power by using it *intelligently, carefully, and judiciously.* The reverse is also true.

Just giving in and going along gives power away. It is almost impossible to perform a task or process well when you disagree with it. People who just give up and go along usually express their power destructively.

How? Coffee and lunch breaks become gripe sessions. Every day is a reminder of the disagreement. Every day the resentment grows. Instead of finding ways to make things work, employees in this situation look for early signs of failure, and tell anyone who listens how awful it is. In short, just giving up and going along can make the entire office screech rather than hum.

If this situation sounds like an experience you've had, treat it as a sign that you have given power away and that you need to begin building and using your power.

Just leaving gives away power. Mr. Sam was fortunate to have guessed right. But a few more facts and dialogue with the physician when his life could be at stake would have been better. Just leaving, either by tuning out or walking out, means that dialogue does not occur, and without dialogue, you can't build your power.

Build your power

Now that we have discussed ways to avoid giving away or losing power, let's move to the topic of building your power. We will examine four ways to build, keep, and use your power.

1. Cultivate dialogue.

Dialogue is the foundation for building power. Cultivating dialogue is as simple as talking to the right people about the right things in the right way at the right time. If your efforts do not cultivate dialogue, take a long hard look at your conversations. One or more of those four things is not right.

You must talk with people at all levels, those who make the rules or control the resources, as well as those who say whether or not you are following the rules or can use the resources. For example, you must talk with people who understand and control the rules on capitation before you can build your power to manage its impact on the practice. And, you must talk with the voice on the phone before you gain the power to minimize the impact of obtaining advance approval for reimbursement of procedures.

When we say "talk with," we mean dialogue, not just trading words. We mean finding out the information and establishing a relationship that allows you to act in your own self-interest in light of the limitations such as budgets, policies, and the written and unwritten "rules of the game".

Suppose Dorothy had continued her dialogue with the Good Witch who sent her down the Yellow Brick Road? What if Dorothy had asked, "Is there another alternative?" or "Can we talk with someone who has met the Wizard?"

OK, the movie may have been shorter and Dorothy would have missed making some wonderful friends. Even more important, without her experiences on the Yellow Brick Road, she may not ever have realized the power she had. It may have taken the crucible of those experiences to refine her power so she could use it. Sometimes, you just gotta' go down the road, and it really helps to have traveling companions who share your quest.

How do you cultivate dialogue? Here's how you might do it if the boss says, "We are going to quit seeing managed care patients because we don't make enough money on them." That's a really great time to say, "Well, we do have a lot of managed care patients, and it could have quite an impact. Could I put some figures together and study it?" The goal in cultivating dialogue is for the conversation to continue, not die.

Chances are, the boss is speaking from emotion and frustration. You may know the financial impact to the penny, and you may know how to improve the profit. But in an unequal power relationship with a frustrated boss, it is a mistake to counter emotions with facts. It's like trying to drown a small fire by dousing it in gasoline. All you get is a hotter fire and maybe even an explosion. You don't get dialogue.

Get the facts and figures. The statement about too little money is partially right, and you are partially right. "Partially right" represents the area for dialogue. Do not, *repeat*, do not tell the boss (or anyone else, for that matter) he or she is partially right. Do not create a dialogue about who's right or wrong. Instead just focus on the issue of revenue versus expenses.

Dialogue, if it can begin, opens with speaking the universal language of any business, dollars. The more you can translate issues into revenue and expense dollars, the greater your chances of dealing successfully with them. This translation does not mean that values and people are not important. It means that you understand the dollar impact of values and people, and puts you in a better position to be responsible to both.

The idea in cultivating dialogue is to continue discussions and to avoid any issues that cause anyone to leave the discussion. The ongoing conversations reveal information, opportunities, and choices that no one saw at the beginning. It's like the journey down the Yellow Brick Road. In the dialogue, everyone discovered strengths and options not seen before. Walking the road in isolated silence and fear overwhelms you with the difficulty of the journey. But, facing the flying monkeys and wicked witches in dialogue with others who share your quest helps each of you survive the journey, deal with the uncertainty and fear, and discover new powers in the process.

2. Examine the premise.

Is it true that the practice does not earn enough money from managed care plans? Examine this premise carefully. Invest a lot of time thinking about the concept behind the statement, as well as the words that make up the statement.

Chances are the premise, as stated, is true. A medical practice cannot thrive under the premise of the tire dealer who bought tires for $35 and sold them for $34. "How do you make money?" he was asked. "I make it on volume," he replied. The trick for the tire dealer (and the medical practice) is to sell for $34 a product that cost a good deal less than $34 to deliver. Look at the words "managed care patients" in the statement. Ask the question another way. "How can we deliver managed care services at an acceptable profit?"

Changing the wording changes the discussion, and that puts you on the road to power. At some point, you may want to say to the boss, "What if we can figure out a way to provide managed care services and keep our costs down?" Who wouldn't go for that changed premise? Power, in this case, begins with questioning the premise to find alternative ways to state the premise. Examining the words may help. For example, the word "patient" implies a relationship that the term "managed care services" does not imply, and that relationship is more costly. That change leads to changed dialogue, with opportunities to change the premise, the details, and obligations while delivering uncompromising quality in health care.

3. Examine the details.

Even if it is true that the practice does not currently

earn enough money from managed care plans, since Americans are rapidly enrolling in such plans, you probably can't refuse to provide managed care services and stay in the health care business. After all, a result of managed care plans is that reimbursing entities, patients, and hospitals have all agreed to a new kind of relationship. They look for providers to join in and deliver, and many are doing so. If your practice does not join in, guess who will have the covered lives!

It could be that the boss's perception of the problem with managed care grows out of trying to continue the old relationships. The boss is not "hearing" everyone else, including patients, asking for a new kind of relationship.

Gather information and find out if the practice treats patients in managed care relationships the same way it treats patients in fee-for-service relationships. If so, the boss is right about the money, but may take another position because of a different understanding of the facts.

J.R., who runs a successful auto service shop, introduced managed care for cars. Knowing that most people want routine repairs at bargain prices, and emergency service when and where needed, he created a service plan to give customers two features hard to find in the same plan. His idea: Paying an annual fee gets your car serviced ahead of customers not in the plan. You get discounts and coupons to apply to repairs, and if you have an emergency within 50 miles of the shop, a mechanic will come immediately to fix your car or tow it. You are charged for parts and the regular labor rates for the repairs, but not for the service run. Paying the annual fee is a "no brainer." J.R. knows how to change relationships to sell managed care and fee-for-service at the same time to the same people.

The new relationships in health care require changes, and not just little changes. Everything in the practice will be affected. Chances are, deep down, everyone knows what must change. Remember, just throwing facts on sparks of frustration can cause a big fire. The universal language of dollars will cause providers to change when it is perceived that change must occur. Consumers will change the way they spend health care dollars when they perceive a value in changing.

All you can do with facts and details is feed them into the dialogue at the time and rate when others will receive them for conversation. Dialogue about the details (such as, we probably won't continue to exist as a practice without providing managed care services) can build the power to re-examine the premise.

4. Examine the obligations.

Examining what you are obliged to do can build the power to examine the details and the premise.

Imagine this situation: Your Medical Records Clerk says, "I spend four hours every day filing documentation of managed care coverage in patient files. The coverage is good for a year, so I also have to remove the old documentation from the file. Is there some way the computer could track whether or not we receive it, and maybe we could store the documents by date?" One hour of data entry could replace four hours of filing every day.

Powerful, costly obligations lead to the questioning of details. How do you keep up with that documentation, and what are some alternatives? The details lead to questioning the assumption that the documents must be filed. Similar questioning of details could lead to similar gains in other areas.

Conclusion

You have power. Use that power many times over, in every area of your responsibilities, and you will affect careers, organizations, and patient care. Power is like tools lying around, just waiting for you to pick them up.

The secret to power is so simple that most people overlook it. Power is reserving the right to choose and act on your own behalf. Every Yellow Brick Road can take you through scary places and to encounters with strange and scary people. So remember, you can retain your power and build it in any situation and in any set of circumstances, unless you give it away.

Begin building power through dialogue. Start with little at stake and leave room to back away for awhile if needed. You can always gain time to think through issues by saying, "I need to think about this and make sure I understand everything involved." Then, think through the premise, details and obligations and discuss them when you are ready to proceed. Well-intentioned and committed people who engage in dialogue can find ways to improve almost any situation.

The process can be great fun after you get used to it. It is especially satisfying to know before you go to sleep at night that you have used your power to take care of yourself. You know then that you can get up in the morning and take care of your organization.

CHAPTER 9

Make your organization succeed

Weeks of rain turned the main street of a frontier town into a quagmire. A person on the sidewalk saw a hat moving in a straight line through the mud toward the end of the street. Picking up the hat, the person was surprised to find a cowpoke underneath, and asked, "Do you need help?"

"No," replied the cowpoke, "I'm doing fine. I'm riding a good horse."

This story, told in the book "A Treasury of American Folklore," contains wisdom for managers in health care. It's easy to look at health care today and see only the quagmire. It's tough to do what the cowpoke did: move with purpose through the muck, confident of your resources and direction, and make your organization succeed.

A medical group succeeds when it carries out its fundamental business proposition of delivering quality medical care. That's a tough challenge. You need the right number of covered lives, acceptable risk pools, proper credentialing, and acceptable "report cards." If you do these things, you are seeing patients and should have enough revenue.

But money coming in is only half of success. You need information processing, registration, medical records, billing, and other operations to operate at maximum efficiency. Then you can pay the bills on time, pay the staff, and earn acceptable profit. Carefully managing the revenue and expense sides of the equation is essential for a medical practice to succeed.

Succeeding is a relative concept. Three years ago, Dr. Godley said, "Let's each see 30 patients a day. Get the patient, the medical record, and the physician in the same room at the same time 90 percent of the time, and this practice succeeds." Now he says "Give us 3,750 covered lives and two nurse practitioners per physician. Get the patient, the medical record, and the provider in the same room at the same time 98 percent of the time. Then, this practice succeeds."

Almost anyone can make an organization succeed when times are great. A few years ago, medical care organizations were almost guaranteed a profit. Physicians set the fees and performed the services they and the patients wanted, and the insurance companies paid the charges. When cost of operations went up, the fees were increased, and higher bills were sent to the payers. It was summertime and the thrivin' was easy.

Well, it's wintertime now, and the thrivin' is not so easy...but it is possible. Succeeding in delivering medical care on financially sound terms can be done if we can see a way through the current muddy conditions of health care. The cowpoke saw an end to the mud. That end for health care is not currently in sight.

As the consultant told a group of practice managers: "Your challenge is to journey from here to there, but there's no 'here' here, there's no 'there' there, and no sure path to follow."

This chapter tells you how to make your organization succeed on that journey.

Making your organization succeed is as simple and as complicated as this: *Identify your organization's critical indicators of success, and talk constantly about how to improve them.* By "constantly," we mean exactly that. There cannot be too much directed, purposeful conversation about efforts to improve those indicators.

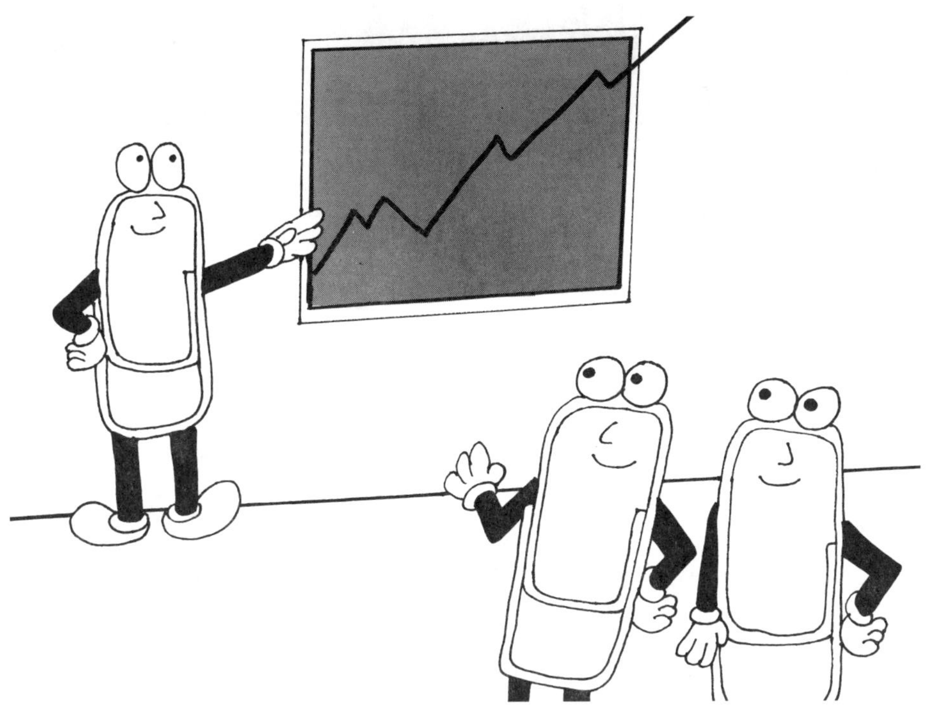

Like the cowpoke, you cannot be deterred by mud and curious strangers. Your goal is to change the conversation in your organization, literally. You want people to quit saying, "Look how deep this mud is!" and start remarking, "Look at our progress through the mud!" Even a little progress causes an interesting transformation. Employees begin to feel power — power over themselves, over the practice, and over the future.

You probably never have to talk about more than five measures of success with any one person. Dealing with more than that bogs you down as a manager in details that the other person should manage. If you are the cowpoke, your list of the top five indicators of success might be:

1. I've got to have cattle ready for sale;
2. Gotta keep my horse healthy;
3. Get this herd closer to trail's end every day;
4. Avoid distractions; and
5. Gotta keep my cowboy hat on.

If you take care of these items, the rest will be easy. Even if they aren't easy, they won't be fatal. But you can't afford to lose sight of those five critical indicators because you are hat deep in the mud.

Identifying the critical measures of success

We advocate continual conversation at work about business topics. One of the points of continual conversation is to identify *changes* in the key indicators of success as conditions change. Conversations with your boss, your employees, and your peers may elate you and may depress you. You may find these people have a clear understanding of some issues and are out to lunch on others.

But it's like Mr. Sam says, "Wherever you are is a good place to start."

Here are several ways to start identifying the indicators and finding out where to begin controlling them.

Review conversations with your boss and physicians.

Take a few hours away from the office. Go to a library, to a quiet outdoor place on a nice day, or to some other place where you can think. Think about conversations with your boss and key physicians when they were upset. Maybe they were concerned with costs, profits, performance...whatever. Write a list of the items as they occur to you. Don't worry about ranking them, just list as many as you can.

Then think about when those same people smiled warmly and expressed satisfaction or happiness with some aspects of life at work. What items made them feel good? Write them on a separate list.

The first list contains some things that key people would apparently like to change. The second list shows what they want continued. The problem is that the emotional content of both unpleasant and pleasant conversations sometimes obscures the specific, controllable issues you would like to identify. Go over your lists in a couple of days. Try to see beyond the feelings, and connect the conversations to specific, controllable activities that affect revenue, expense, and quality of care.

Now, rank the items in the order of their impact on the organization's success. What we would like to find are people-controllable items that cost little or no additional money to deal with. They can be improved simply by doing things differently. Which item could produce the largest improvement? That's the top priority. Which could produce the next largest improvement, and so on. Pretty soon, you have candidates for the five most critical indicators of success.

Use continuous improvement techniques.

Another way to begin identifying the indicators is to use continuous improvement techniques. American industry, and the automotive industry in particular, used them to help regain competitive edges. Techniques such as brainstorming, cause-and-effect diagrams, and Pareto analysis give you powerful tools for starting conversations about improvements. Colleges and universities generally offer classes on using these techniques in their Continuing Education Departments or in their Schools of Business. There also are many books available on Total Quality Management/Continuous Quality Improvement.

Use MGMA resources.

The MGMA Library Resource Center maintains statistical studies of health care delivery factors such as productivity. These studies can help identify key indicators of success for medical practices. In addition, some studies include benchmarks you can use to compare your practice with others.

Use a combination of these techniques, or others you know, to develop a preliminary list of the critical indicators of success for the organization. Then, list the handful of critical success indicators for departments, and the most important areas of coordination among departments.

Next, begin talking with people about these factors as a way to verify the lists. Talk with your boss, with your employees, and with your peers. Then you can begin in earnest to talk constantly, constantly, about improving performance in the areas that matter most.

Know thy boss (and converse with same)

The changes in health care over the past few years include changes in how to identify your boss. It used to be simpler, and the relationships were clearer. While medical group managers have often been in the uneasy position of having multiple bosses, usually those bosses had a lot in common, because they were all physicians. Now your bosses may include combinations of physicians, administrators, corporate managers, and boards.

Identify your boss(es) by making a list and checking it twice. If you leave a boss off your list, expect a lump of coal. Identify your boss(es) and talk with him/her/it/them. For now, let's make things simple and assume that Dr. Godley is your boss. "Dr. Godley, here is a summary of the five current most critical indicators of the practice's success that I manage:

1. Labor costs as a percentage of revenue;
2. Overtime costs;
3. Percentage of overall administrative costs;
4. Patient flow; and
5. Medical records cost/benefit.

"Can we talk about them?"

This list is from a hypothetical private practice, and predates capitation, which uses a different set of indicators. The capitation list would probably include issues such as the number of covered lives, adverse selection ratio, capitation rates, and others.

Most medical groups deal with what has been called "the schizophrenic mixture of fee-for-service and managed care patients." The indicators of success must address *your* group in your location with your patients and your problems. But the concept is the same regardless of the setting: identify what factors are most important, and get everyone in the organization talking about those things.

Create a one-page summary with a paragraph on each item. The paragraphs outline where the organization is now with each item, as well as where you think the organization should be in 1-18 months. The period depends on the length of time it takes to change the particular item. Spend a lot of time on this summary. Make sure you can support it with facts and figures. Done properly and with the right issues, this summary starts the needed discussions.

Note: Some conversations may become heated, especially if the facts and figures contradict anyone's beliefs about the practice. This can be unpleasant — just like taking strong medicine can be unpleasant — but the end result is worth the intermediate pain.

Continue the conversations with your boss on a regular schedule. Some bosses like to go ahead and write meeting dates on the calendar. Others resist scheduling, but like you to catch them every month. There is nothing wrong with calling the boss periodically and saying, "Could we meet for a few minutes and talk about my department?" Initiate these conversations, if your boss has not already started them with you.

These regular conversations with your boss about the five most critical indicators of success give you three forms of invaluable feedback:

1. They help you know if you are using your resources to address the most critical needs of the practice, as seen by those who control the practice;

2. They tell you if management is willing to address those needs; and

3. They tell you if management is willing to let you help.

Negative feedback on any one of the three probably means that you will not be allowed as active a role as you would like in the organization. The organization may succeed, and you may help by working harder and longer, but you will have to go along for whatever ride the boss decides to take.

A real advantage to these conversations is that it helps bosses — particularly physicians — see new possibilities, gain perspective, and overcome fear of losing control of the practice. Your analyses and plans for managing the most critical aspects of the practice could make a difference in their future plans: to sell, merge, expand, contract, or stay the same.

Some physicians have made bad decisions out of fear because they felt they had no options. Your goal is to give them options when the MegaHealths — whose managers understand finance and the psychology of fear better than they understand medicine — come calling.

Talk with your people

You will come away from the conversations with your bosses with a fairly clear understanding of their vision, their priorities, and the level of support you have for taking action. As the person in the middle, you get to translate these issues into effective action by your staff.

Talk with each of them about the three-to-five most critical indicators of success they manage. That is how you begin reshaping the organization for the realities of changing health care.

Your task is to help reshape the organization and bring it into the new health care game as a strong player. The survival of your organization, or the conditions for joining a larger one, may well depend on how you translate the top five critical indicators of success into action by staff.

Suppose Ms. Smart calls Joan and says, "Joan, I'm meeting with each of the department managers to talk about our challenges in the next 18 months. I want to talk with you about improving the three-to-five most critical indicators of success in Medical Records. Some of the things on my quick list are:

- timely pulling of charts;
- correct filing of documents;
- obtaining documentation from the physicians; and
- reducing labor costs.

Let's meet next Wednesday and talk about it. I would like your ideas. We'll create a list, make sure that the physicians are comfortable with it, and then get to work. I want us to concentrate on changes we can make at little or no cost."

Done in an open and non-threatening manner, conversations like this are almost guaranteed to improve operations.

The willingness of employees to engage in such conversations tells managers whether employees will help restructure the organization or will resist change. Managers have more influence on *people* than on any other factor that determines an organization's success. Huge improvements are possible by working with people to change what they do and how they do it, without spending significant amounts of money. When people see the possibility of making things better, they usually become happier and more productive.

After Ms. Smart talks with Joan, Joan needs to have similar conversations with each Medical Records employee, asking them about the most critical indicators of success for a Medical Records employee, When Joan and the employees agree on these indicators, talking about them and controlling them becomes easier.

So Joan initiates the following conversation with Alice, one of the Medical Records assistants:

"Alice, one of the most important things we can do in this department, as I see it, is to make sure people don't have to wait for charts. What do you think?"

"I think you're right," replies Alice.

"Name some other things that are really important," asks Joan.

Alice thinks for a few seconds and replies, "Inserting the necessary documents and refiling the medical records as quickly as possible, unless there is a referral."

They are on the right track. Through questions and answers, they will come up with a good list. Then they need to talk about improving performance in those areas.

Often, the employees who do the jobs know more about them than anyone else. The idea is to get those people involved in achieving many small incremental gains. If employees can identify two documents routinely included in medical records that can be eliminated, the savings over time can be significant. If they can quantify the time it takes to locate medical records stalled at someone's desk when they should be circulating, the people and processes that create the delays can be worked on.

Joan must obtain the support of her bosses before making any major changes. If the impact is significant, her task is to package the request in terms of the improvements it will produce, and to present it at the proper time. We don't mean to leave you with the impression that only items of major impact should be considered. If the impact is significant, that's great, but small incremental gains can add up. After all, you are probably more likely to find 50 ways to save $10 than one way to save $500. The idea is to get everyone thinking and talking about the factors that produce improvements.

Ms. Smart should talk with each person reporting to her, and those people should do likewise. In each case the idea is to target the greatest gains in each person's area of responsibility, and to establish goals.

Regular conversations with employees about improving the five most critical indicators of success will change the content of conversations in the workplace. When that occurs, people's thought processes change. Employees begin to think and talk about making steady progress. The progress can be quantified and reported.

Feedback is important. Reporting the gains that result from employees' efforts *to the employees who made the effort* tells them what to continue and what to change.

People who see that their efforts make a difference usually increase their efforts. They feel power, and they exercise it to make the organization succeed and make their jobs more interesting and secure.

Two words of caution apply:

First, don't micro-manage your people. Micro-managing bogs you down in the operational details, robs people of the opportunity to perform, and shuts down suggestions from the people who know the most about the task. After all, you don't do the nitty gritty work of medical records every day, just as Joan does not do the nitty gritty work of pulling charts, filing documents, and replacing charts. Gains come from people who do the work daily and think about ways to improve it.

Second, be ready to replace employees who will not engage in the conversations and assume responsibility for improvements. Make sure you have your superior's support for this.

Give those employees two or three opportunities to cooperate. Write out objectives and completion dates, and document their performance. Use performance as the basis for rewarding employees or suggesting that specific employees need to search for other opportunities.

If an employee does not cooperate in the process, the organization simply cannot afford to keep that employee. If you have to terminate someone's employment, make sure you comply with applicable standards for documentation, counseling, and non-discrimination based on race, age, gender, disability, etc.

It *is* possible to discharge employees in bureaucratic organizations such as public agencies. The trick is to learn the rules and play by them patiently and methodically. Using the resources of a competent labor attorney or human resources consultant is worth the cost if you are not sure about the process.

You'll thank me when you're older

Employees who really want to affect their futures will thank you for the conversations and will throw themselves eagerly into the process of improving the critical indicators of success. Help them improve their performance, as measured against the goals related to the indicators of success.

Be sure to talk with peers about the five most important indicators of success that require coordination among departments.

An observation consultants often make is: "In some companies, the only thing employees have in common is that the same computer-generated signature is on all the paychecks. There is no evidence of a common mission, a shared understanding of each department's contribution to that mission, and a clear coordination among the key managers in carrying out that mission."

The data-processing manager in one such health care organization observed that "Employees don't care about learning to use the registration system. Why, we've put in improvements for registering patients, enhanced them, and then replaced them...and the registration staff never even knew the features were there." Suppose that data-processing manager had talked with her peer, the manager of registration, in advance of spending the thousands of dollars on the improvements?

The goal in talking with peers is to change the conversations and thought processes among same-level employees. Make your organization succeed by talking constantly with peers about the five most important issues of coordination among departments. That's five issues in total among all managers, not five issues with each manager.

What if Joan made this phone call:

"Emily, this is Joan in Medical Records. Can we spend a few minutes talking about the coordination between my staff and your medical assistants? I believe you and I can eliminate most of the yelling sessions about waiting for charts."

After Joan and Emily made progress in coordinating the efforts of their two departments, suppose Emily called the data-processing manager, saying, "I'm not sure we are making the best use of the data-processing support. Could you have someone talk us through the features, functions and capabilities as a check on our understanding of it?"

You get the picture. Similar phone calls to other key managers will slowly change the conversations, thought processes, and working relationships between departments. The approach must always be: "I want to make sure my department coordinates with your department in improving operations. I need your help, and I want to help you. After all, we are in this together and if things don't improve, we'll all be out of work."

Those conversations with peers can be the first step toward achieving huge incremental gains. Your goal: An absolute commitment of all key managers to coordinate efforts in improving performance.

Again, some words of caution. Some managers may respond suspiciously. However, if there are valid areas for coordination and discussion, your challenge is to present them to other managers in terms of their own self-interests. If they feel you are trying to gain power over them, they will resist.

Some final suggestions:

1. You should be able to quantify the critical indicators of success, and you must be able to measure progress toward the goals you set. Without quantifying, the best you can do is to bet your good, warm feeling against someone else's bad, cold feeling. (If you bet yours against the bosses', want to guess who wins?)

2. Evaluate performance based on each employee's contributions to improving the critical indicators of success, and give compliments, perks, ratings, and raises on the same basis.

If you do not focus on performance, your rewards will negate everything you are trying to accomplish. For example, just give the same raise to the employee who stretches three hours of work into eight hours as you give to a high-performing employee. That'll change the thought process and conversation all right, but not in the desired manner.

Sometimes we are stuck with policies that stink. The boss(es) said, "Everybody gets *x* percent raise." If it stinks, tell employees that you yourself may not prefer that approach, but you support company policy, and you will reward them in other ways when you are able. Recognition, cross-training, seminars, and an occasional few hours off or extra time for lunch when they get ahead of schedule can really help. Just make sure you can do it without causing problems for yourself and the productive employees.

3. Practice benevolent intolerance for everything that does not directly improve a critical indicator of success.

Let's look at two examples where benevolent intolerance is needed.

Example One: The data-processing manager and the registration manager have been wasting time and resources blaming each other for the problems with the system. Benevolent intolerance suggests having them in for a joint visit, which begins something like this:

"Let me talk with both of you about acceptable and unacceptable work behavior. Acceptable is working together to solve the problem. Unacceptable at this point is for there to be even one more accusation. You work it out, or I will work it out for you. I want to meet with you again Friday and hear your plan."

Example Two: After this conversation, one of the managers just didn't get the point. You happen by a working session between the two managers, and you hear the registration manager say, "If you and your programmers weren't so busy trying to control my department, you could create a system that works."

Benevolent intolerance suggests this conversation with that person within the next day or so:

"I overheard your comment to the data-processing manager. The job of registration manager requires working well with data processing. The job will be done right, and that is not negotiable. Someone *will* do it right. I sincerely hope you are the person who does it, but that is up to you.

"Here's how I want your conversations to occur... (etc., etc.)

"You have one month to show me you can do it. I want you to do it, but it is your choice."

Put the details in a memorandum, establish a follow-up date, and hold the person accountable.

Benevolent intolerance emphasizes benevolence. There's no reason to be angry with anyone. There is no reason to question if they care. There is no reason to try to squeeze the desired behavior out of them. Those actions lead to time-consuming discussions and sometimes even to legal charges.

On the other hand, there is plenty of reason to be descriptive. Describe what the job requires, describe what the person did, describe the changes that must be made and when they must be made. Then the person either chooses to do it, or chooses not to do it.

Conclusion

Making your organization succeed is as simple and as complicated as talking constantly about the five most critical indicators of success. Talk about them with your boss, with your employees, and with your peers. That's how managers in health care gain control over the issues that determine their futures.

The concept is simple, but it is hard work to change people's thought processes and conversations.

Let's say you succeed in this endeavor, and that the approach succeeds so well that the physicians get a much higher offer for the practice than the offer they got 18 months ago. They decide to take the money, and they politely thank you for making them a lot of money. Do you suppose MegaHealth has a place for someone who knows how to make an organization succeed? And if you don't want to work for MegaHealth, we heard Dr. Preen may have to sell his practice unless he can find someone to restructure it. You might be in a good position to negotiate!

CHAPTER 10

Clarify your values

Chapter 10–Clarify your values

We intend this chapter to help you become more conscious of values, and their effects on performance and relationships at work. In the process, we will ask you to examine and clarify your values. Knowing your values clearly is essential to taking care of yourself so you can take care of your organization.

It can be quite difficult to define "values," but for the purpose of this chapter we can safely say that, whatever your values are, they are indicated by the way you invest your time, energy, and resources.

Values drive human behavior. All day, every day, all of us act on our values. Speeding up to make a caution light and save time represents one value. Braking for the caution light at the cost of time represents a different value. Yogurt contains less fat, and that is valuable to some people. But chocolate fudge tastes just sooooooooo good — another value. Your decisions and actions and choices depend on what you value most in the situation.

Values can get complicated. For example, most people want to recycle, but the "rules" are confusing. Do you say "paper" or "plastic" when the check-out clerk asks you about bags? Using paper bags kills trees. And yet trees are a renewable resource. Using plastic bags saves trees, but may pollute. And though some plastic bags are recyclable, how much plastic is actually recycled? Or how much paper, for that matter? Do we have enough facts to make a good decision?

We cannot escape making decisions and choices. Our decisions will be based on our values, and our values will be based on...what? Fact? Myth? Emotion? Culture? Instinct? Reason? All of those factors and perhaps many more. The point: Developing a good, clear picture of our values might help us understand *why* we choose the things we do, and might help us avoid those frustrating situations where all the choices seem to conflict with our values.

Values and work

Whether to use paper or plastic bags is one thing. The values we deal with at work present us with tougher choices and personally higher stakes. Values affect relationships with bosses, co-workers, and patients. Values affect the quality of care and the efficiency of the organization.

Lauree ran into some of the tough issues related to values on her first day as Dr. Godley's Medical Assistant. She finally found time for a break in the middle of the morning, and she really needed it. She was not a happy camper. "I've never seen anything like it," she complained to Jeannie. "That man expects everything to be perfect. It's assembly-line medicine, the way he runs from patient to patient. He even told me to move faster because he wants to improve his utilization review numbers. I'm pooped."

Jeannie had worked there five years, including two as Dr. Godley's Medical Assistant. "It's tough staying up with him," she replied. "You really have to know what you are doing, and he wants you to think constantly about how to do it better. It can wear you out. But if you want to learn a lot about good medical care, he's your man."

This response surprised Lauree. She replied, "But he talked about making sure we saw all of his patients without wasting one second. When we got ahead of his schedule, he even volunteered to see patients of other physicians. I think all he sees is the cash. His values are all twisted around."

"I felt the same way at first," Jeannie said. "Then I noticed that the patients love him. Did you see any of his patients looking displeased?"

"Well, no..."

"See? That's my impression too," Jeannie responded.

"So how does he practice assembly-line medicine and make patients like it?" asked Lauree.

"Maybe you should ask him," Jeannie suggested.

At that moment Dr. Godley stuck his head in the door and said, "Lauree, do you mind starting again now? I think we can finish early."

After the last patient, including two scheduled for other physicians, Lauree asked, "Dr. Godley, how do you do it? You see patients so quickly, but they all look happy."

He said, "Let's get some coffee and chat for a minute." They walked to the break room and found a quiet table. "One reason I try to stay ahead of schedule," Dr. Godley continued, "is because that gives me extra time for patients who really need it *and* for talking with my staff.

"As to your question, I hope the patients know that I care about them and that they will receive the best medical care I can deliver," he continued. "It's true I tend to work quickly. But you know what? Over the years, I've noticed that patients seem to shop around for a primary care doctor until they find one whose style they like. Many of my patients are busy people themselves, and they don't like to be kept waiting. My patients seem to place a high value on 'accessibility.' They don't call unnecessarily, and they don't come in for hand-holding and counseling.

"There are lots of exceptions, of course. But if you compare my practice with, say, Dr. Foster's, you really can tell a difference. Dr. Foster is quiet and caring and tender, just a marvelous human being, and her practice attracts a lot of patients who want to see her for emotional support. They trust her, and they ask her for advice on all kinds of things."

Dr. Godley chuckled and said, "Some of her patients hate it when I cover for Dr. Foster. I just don't have her style. They find me too practical, too mechanical, compared to her."

Jeannie saw Lauree again several weeks later, and asked how she was doing with Dr. Godley. "I'm still running my legs off, but it's getting better. You know, maybe it's not just the money when he talks about improving the numbers," she said. Lauree paused, and then said, "Medicine really seems to be his life. I think he would see patients for nothing if that is what it took for him to practice medicine. I think he looks to the numbers just to make sure that he sees all the people who need to be seen. Getting ahead on routine examinations lets him spend more time when it is really needed."

Values and relationships

We will resist the urge to tie up this story neatly and with a happy ending. Like everyone else in the health care business, Lauree struggles with the forces that are shaping our futures. We will leave the finishing of Lauree's and Dr. Godley's story to your imagination. Instead we will make these points about values:

- Several people can view the same situation and reach radically different conclusions about the values that drive human behavior. One person's "good medicine" is another person's "assembly-line medicine." It depends on the conscious and unconscious values each brings to the definition.

In the previous story, Lauree's first impression of Dr. Godley was pretty unfavorable. And there seems to be no doubt that Dr. Godley had driven off other staff people and other patients in the past. But the staff and patients who stayed with him think he is terrific.

- It is necessary to clarify your values in order to work effectively in changing situations. For Lauree to continue working with Dr. Godley, she would profit from not judging him hastily. Instead she should extend the benefit of the doubt toward him while she tries to gain a wider perspective on his values. But even more important, she would benefit from a serious effort to understand her *own* values.

Through good luck or bad, Lauree is now working side by side with a person whose outlook on some important issues may be quite different from hers. The two of them must find ways to forge a working relationship. And let's face it, they are not equals in this setting. Lauree is faced with a choice: to learn and grow from this challenging situation and this relationship, or to withdraw from it. In simple words, she can expand or she can contract as a person. She can throw herself into it, or run away from it.

Lauree actually has an entire range of responses she can make:

- openness;
- accommodation;
- tolerance;
- civility;
- stand-offishness;
- disdain; or
- active hostility.

Over time, if her responses keep coming from the bottom part of the list, conflict is inevitable. Conflict would spill over into poor performance, with two consequences: (1) she would be miserable; and (2) since Dr. Godley does not tolerate poor performance, she would probably lose her job.

Keeping a job where your values are constantly under assault is not a good thing. But the real point is to be sure of what your values really *are*. Only then can you decide what is worth fighting for.

As an aside, it is interesting to note that Lauree does not, in the practical world, have much chance of making Dr. Godley's values correspond with hers. And, of course, Dr. Godley faces the same situation in his relationship with Lauree.

- It is easier to criticize the values of others than to learn from them and do the hard work of clarifying one's own values with new information and different perspectives. Luckily, Lauree's conversation with Dr. Godley, along with Jeannie's ideas, showed her another way of looking at the situation. From that angle, Lauree's value of providing the best possible care to the most patients was supported, not contradicted.

Like all of us, Lauree has to deliver medical care in ways that are possible, which may not be how we would do things if money and time were not issues.

Ending this story by saying: "And they lived happily ever after" would send the wrong message. Real life usually does not lead to that result. In real life, we experience values in the middle, in the shades of grey, not black and white. We operate in areas where values collide. We can view those engagements as opportunities for growth through dialogue, or we can view them as the boundaries of a battle.

Values and zones of comfort

Like most of us, Dr. Godley works best when he feels "comfortable." Being "comfortable" means our needs are being met physically, emotionally, and spiritually. Just what that means is a highly individual definition, determined by our personal values.

Where we invest our time, energy, and resources indicates our values, our zones of comfort; each of us may have several zones. Dr. Godley is neither a self-giving humanitarian nor a money-grubbing, do-it-by-the-numbers, revenue-producing-and-cost-cutting machine.

Dr. Godley needs to feel that his efforts make him comfortable. His current definition of comfort includes time for reflecting about the meaning of life, intimacy with his family, new cars, long vacations, a nice home, and a solid financial portfolio. Being comfortable in those zones frees him to heal, care, and contribute to the advancements in medical science, which represents yet another zone of comfort.

Lauree's current definition of comfort at work includes more time with people, a less hectic pace, and delivering good medical care as she see it. These are important to her emotional and spiritual comfort. Like her boss, being comfortable frees her to heal, care and contribute at her level in delivering health care. All of us, like Dr. Godley and Lauree, invest ourselves in the attempt to become "comfortable." Lauree's conflict with Dr. Godley's values stems from her discomfort with the way he treated people — namely Lauree herself, the patients, and other physicians. This conflict caused her to say "his values are all twisted around."

Let's shift from Lauree and Dr. Godley to our own places of work and the decisions we face. How can we treat patients as human beings while reducing costs? How do we spend less time with them and get them to like it? We have three people too many, but don't want anyone to lose a job. There just has to be a way to tell Dr. Preen that his condescending treatment of the staff causes turnover. Do I take the position with Megahealth and move my family?

We have to face decisions involving conflicting values every day. Without being assured of reaching the destination, we set out on paths that we expect will lead us to comfort. We are more likely to achieve comfort in the physical, emotional, and spiritual zones when we are conscious of our values, when we clarify them through critical examination, and when we commit ourselves deliberately and consciously to behaviors consistent with our values.

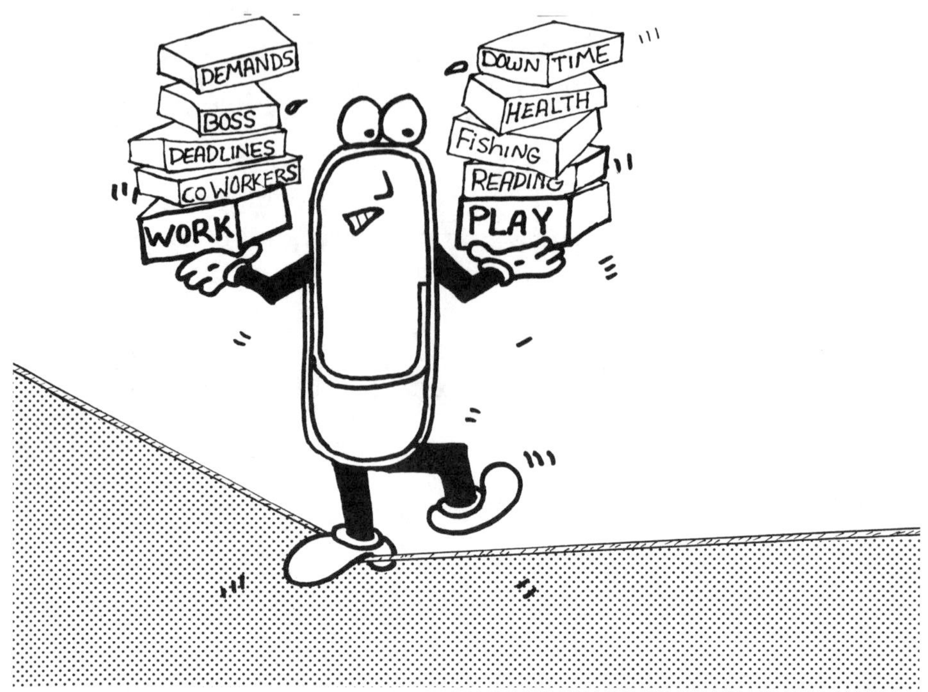

Clarifying your values

What does it mean to clarify your values? And how do you go about doing it?

Clarifying your values means: (1) defining or verifying your core values to make sure you are willing to bet your future on them; (2) examining how your behavior matches or does not match your core values; (3) examining how your organization's behavior complements or conflicts with your core values; (4) creating partnerships instead of conflict with those whose values differ from yours so you can learn from them; and (5) creating new ways to abide by your core values in changed circumstances.

Just to be clear, let's point out specifically that "clarifying your values" does not mean simply adopting values that are handy for the moment, or compromising your values, or rationalizing that you have no choice.

In the remainder of this chapter we will take these five items and relate them to a few real-life illustrations and observations about why it is important for people to understand and work in harmony with their values. Then we will discuss "how" to clarify values.

Core values, decisions, organizations

Had Tim, unemployed in Kansas, spent more time beforehand defining and verifying his core values, he may have avoided that situation, or perhaps he might have chosen a different risk. But his value system required the perceived security of working within a large organization. Tim needs that kind of support structure, and he likes being surrounded by lots of people. His actions were consistent with his values. However, had he more carefully examined his core values and those of the organization he worked for, he may well have uncovered inconsistences that would have given him serious reason to question whether to move.

Tim saw no other organization to join, so he went to Kansas, without examining the organization's behavior to see whether it was consistent with his core values. As he filed for unemployment compensation, he mumbled to himself, "I wish I had spent more time questioning whether the company was willing to give me as much commitment as I gave it."

Values, conversation, partnership

A happier example: Lauree moved from confrontation to conversation, not battle. She confronted her differences with Dr. Godley internally by acknowledging them and her strong feelings. Then she engaged him in conversation and tried to look for common ground.

When we left their story, she and Dr. Godley were talking, not fighting. Their working relationship had the potential for an effective partnership in which the professional behavior of each could be consistent with their own personal core values. The core values of each individual included conversation instead of conflict, and that made the difference.

Since we cannot "freeze" reality at any point in time, we have to adjust to change and to changing realities constantly. Lauree's core values provided her a foundation for discussions and a partnership with someone whose values differed from hers.

Telling people to set aside their differences and to look for common ground can be a tall order. Labels like "compromise," "wishy-washy," and "uncommitted" lurk in the background, ready to be applied. But think about it: Those who are secure in their core values can examine and discuss differing values without fear.

The minimum benefit of such conversations is the reconfirmation of one's core values. ("Yep, I was right the first time.") But often the benefit will be a clarification from learning new points of view. On the other hand, uncertainty about core values can expose one to the possibility that differing values will displace rather than teach.

Solid core values permit a number of alternatives for acting on them. After all, if the core value is to take care of patients, you don't quit providing care just because you think the physician may be rushing things a bit. An alternative is to discover how to provide the kind of care the patients want, and then to deliver it efficiently. *That* is what Lauree was learning from her conversations with Dr. Godley.

Values and dramatic changes

One of the authors recently went to a barrier island in hope of a week of lazy days walking on the beach and staring reflectively over the water. A hurricane changed the situation and gave him an unexpected opportunity to clarify his values. Safety became more valuable than staying on the beach, and comfort meant leaving the island. The remaining days of vacation at a lake lodge still accomplished what he needed, lazy days and reflection.

Core values don't change simply because the situation changes. A week on the beach is not quite a core value, but taking time for reflection, and living "the examined life" are core values. The behavior changed from walking on the beach to strolling by the lake, but the underlying value did not change.

Similarly, a committed physician would not stop seeing patients because the economics change. Dr. Foster, the associate Dr. Godley mentioned to Lauree, may be exposed to a reduction of income in the future because her values as reflected in her style of practice don't "pay off" under the realities of managed care. She may have some tough choices to make. The key point: If taking care of people is a central part of her life, if it is something so strong in her make-up that she literally defines herself in that way, then one of the choices she *doesn't* have is to stop seeing patients.

Sometimes dramatic changes lead to new values because the new situation is so radically different. For example, many physicians who valued their independence five years ago now value it less due to the changing economics of medical practice.

Like Dr. Godley, physicians who used to value spending time with patients when the insurance companies would pay for it, now value efficiency in seeing patients. The only way to continue practicing medicine may be for everyone involved in patient care to make changes in the way they invest time in patients and related activities. Those changes generate the cash flow necessary to continue in medicine. Without the cash, physicians might not be able to see patients...and that is a situation totally unacceptable to their core values.

As mentioned previously, the "what" of clarifying your values involves five things: Defining or verifying your core values, examining how your behavior matches your core values, examining how your organization's behavior matches your core values, creating partnerships instead of battle, and creating new ways to carry out your core values in changed circumstances. Addressing these issues helps you progress toward emotional, physical, and spiritual comfort when the path is not clear.

How to clarify your values

Now, the "how" of clarifying your values. Clarifying your values can be really hard work, but the approach is fairly simple. Ask and answer six questions:

1. What do you want?
2. Does your effort help you get what you want?
3. Are the tradeoffs worth it?
4. Are you decorating a box?
5. How do you act under pressure?
6. Do your values make others uncomfortable?

As you may suspect, these questions provide a lifetime of self-examination. You will always be caught in the middle, between the clear question and less-clear answers that come with any set of circumstances.

Let's examine each of these questions in detail.

What do you want?

Most us are as clear as Dr. Godley about our values — absolutely clear on some things and absolutely vague on other things. "I want to hang onto this job until I reach retirement." "I want to keep this job until something better comes along." "I want to make a difference in lives." "I want time for family, gardening, and reading." "I want to pay for my kids' college education." "I want to enjoy work." "I want to chuck it all and live a simple life on a subsistence farm." "I want to get away from the stress and anger." "I want to ___________________." Look deep down inside and fill in the blank with what you really want.

While you are looking, reflect on the difference between processes and results. Keeping your current job may be a process. Time for family, gardening, and reading is a result. Treating a process as a result can cause you to lose perspective and hurt yourself. For Lauree, trying stubbornly to stay up with Dr. Godley may be a process doomed to failure. It can lead to disenchantment with medicine, with the job, and even to personal health problems. Walking stubbornly on the beach during a hurricane does not lead to lazy days and reflection. If the process does not produce the desired result, maybe you should consider changing the process.

Clarify what you want out of work and out of life. Make a list of each. Use the list as a landmark over the next 18 months. Without a landmark, you don't know if your efforts get you closer or take you farther away from your goal. You could end up like the classic frustrated, miserable person who complains about being unhappy. Asked, "What do you want?", the person replies, "Not this!" There is no ability to define "This is what I want" and to invest intelligently toward achieving it.

Does your effort help you get what you want?

Investing time, energy, and resources without clarifying values guarantees frustration. Stated bluntly, working 10 hours a day and taking work home in the vague hope that Dr. Godley will reward you and that things will work out sets you up for disappointment.

Define the desired payoff and obtain commitment from those who control it before investing your effort. If you do not get the assurances you want, adjust your investment to equal the agreements you can get. Failure to adjust what you give to what you get can lead to problems such as: You may get surprises like the one Tim got; others may take advantage of you; and you may feel out of touch with yourself because your best energies go to things you don't really like.

Physicians have to change the way they spend time with patients to carry out their core values of providing quality medical care *and* building a solid economic foundation for the practice. As Dr. Godley told Lauree, those goals are not mutually exclusive. Similarly, you also may have to adjust your behavior or refine your values to achieve what you want. And, like most people, you may prefer not to change.

If your investment in your current job does not help you get what you want, you have other options than quitting. For example, you can try, try really hard, to change what's happening at work.

One manager called a staff meeting and started with this statement: "We are so busy with meetings and projects that we have lost sight of our goals. Our goals are simple. Deliver quality medical care as measured by utilization review, increase revenue by five percent, and decrease costs by five percent. Let's look at plans for this week, and cancel everything that does not measurably contribute to those goals."

That kind of acid test from time to time can radically change the investment of time, energy, and resources. It also changes the level of satisfaction or frustration. If such an acid test does not give you and your organization options for substantive change, *then* you may want to think seriously about changing organizations.

Don't be too quick to change because of uncertainty and insecurity. People in health care will just have to live with uncertainty and insecurity for a period of time. Therefore, we don't believe that all ships taking on water are like the Titanic. Nor do we believe that a ship will sink just because it has a hole in the hull. Most health care ships leak these days. But, if the captains will not allow you to patch the hole and pump out the water, don't spend your time rearranging the deck chairs.

People in health care want to take care of patients, help heal bodies and minds, and help others live productive lives. To act on those values, it may be necessary to radically restructure organizations, change the way they do their jobs, or even leave for a new job. If your current situation does not help you act out your values, and if it cannot be changed, you may find it necessary to do something else, based on what you know about yourself after a thorough examination of your values and options.

Are the tradeoffs worth it?

A tradeoff in terms of values means you give up something or invest something to get the benefits of one of the four classical motivators of human behavior: opportunity, security, prestige, or autonomy. Employment usually requires trading off your time and your energy, perhaps your comfort, and to some extent your values, to obtain one or more of those four.

Most of us easily understand the time and energy tradeoffs. The tradeoffs of comfort and of values may be less clear. Employers generally want loyalty to the *organization's* values from employees, and those values can range from major issues to minor preferences. As a common example, if the boss likes conservative clothing, employees tend to dress conservatively, even when their own tastes are different. The dress code is not a major problem with most employees. But as the issues become more important, employment may mean keeping quiet about your values, and it can mean pressure to change your values or act in contradiction to them.

Deep down, at night before you go to sleep, is what you get worth what you give up? The answer comes from your values, whether you have clarified them or not, and whether you are conscious of them or not.

Are you decorating a box?

John Steinbeck observes in his book "Sweet Thursday" that people who find themselves living in a box usually decorate it. His comment referred to a young woman who lived inside an abandoned steam boiler. She glued fabric to the walls so she would not feel trapped in a box, but instead would feel that she lived free, in an airy room with curtains and windows.

Steinbeck's observation parallels another observation in the book "Corporate Cultures." People take on the value system of their corporate sub-group. Thus, tobacco industry CEO's can look straight at a camera and say, "Nicotine is not addictive." Employees can say of an abusive boss, "He's not really mean, that's just his way of testing people." People can say of a situation they hate, "The benefits here are terrific."

Are you decorating a box? Do the title, the salary, the benefits, the perceived security, and other perks persuade you to feel that it is something else? People sometimes become very comfortable in routines that can destroy them. If your job requires you to give yourself to activities that go against your value system, the familiar box can become a coffin.

Sometimes, however, you need to decorate a box to make the best of a bad situation for a period of time. That may be the only way to stand it while you plan and work your way carefully toward something else.

On the other hand, sometimes you need to rip the decorations off and look at the box as it is. Tim accepted the position of Director of Human Resources in one of MegaHealth's Kansas hospitals. The job seemed right, the money was right, and the working relationship with the Administrator felt right. But in his first staff meeting, Tim watched in shock as the charming, friendly Administrator who had interviewed him turned into a raving, screaming, abusive demagogue.

Tim is not yet unemployed, but he is looking for a new job. He ripped down the decorations that he, Tim, had put up to make him feel as though his situation was tenable. Yes, the Administrator had "sold" him, and he had bought it. But Tim learned an important lesson about values — values come from within, not from rubber stamping someone else's.

Tim and his family now have the goal of saving the equivalent of one year's income, and they have scaled back their consumption. "Never again," says Tim, "will I be in the position where financial necessity dictates that I must tolerate abuse." He has clarified his values.

How do you act under pressure?

Mark Twain told a story about a group of travelers in the late 1800's whose stagecoach broke down in an area where they did not feel safe. The pressure of the situation gave them few options. One of the travelers, feeling the pressure, jumped on a horse and rode off madly in all directions at once to look for help. He got nowhere fast.

How do *you* act under pressure? Let's say you are in the middle of a computer conversion; you have to prepare a special set of financial statements; reports are due for the board meeting; a relative is ill; your car did not start; three employees are absent; half the phones don't work; and the boss says, "We have to bid on managed care contract for 15,000 covered lives by one week from today, so drop everything and get to work on it!"

That's pressure!

Pressure reveals our value system and gets it out in the open so we can examine it. What do you do under pressure? What are your gut responses? As with Mark Twain's travelers, our options under pressure are relatively few. Our reactions under pressure represent values that powerfully affect our futures.

Some managers under pressure simply give up trying to affect the future and wait for it to arrive. Others try everything that comes along, substituting activity for accomplishment. Many use "You should have known..." and other forms of blame, to cover their inadequacies. A few want to fire everybody and hire some "really good people." Still others check out the latest theories from the current management guru and send everybody to a seminar. Some managers read everything and digest little.

But some managers gather information, sort through the issues, understand their implications, outline a sound course of action, and work carefully with the bosses and the staff to take care of themselves and their organization. These are the most effective managers. Your gut-level "feeling" reactions to pressure determine whether you will be among that group.

Your actions when the pressure cooker steams, when the fat is in the fire, when the heat is on, when the swamp is full of alligators — choose your own metaphor — tell you and others a great deal about your values. If you react with panic, so will your staff. If you react by complaining and moaning, so will your staff. If you react calmly, so will the staff. Look at what you do under pressure. If your behavior does not get the results you want, clarify your values and act differently.

Do your values make others uncomfortable?

"Here, see if you can peel this thing for me," said Ron, Ms. Smart's spouse, as he handed her the not-quite-ripe banana he had struggled with for several minutes. Ms. Smart took the banana, turned it stem end down, peeled it effortlessly from the "wrong" end, and smugly handed it back to him.

"If you ever wonder why people sometimes think you are a smart-aleck, that's why," said Ron. "It really makes people feel stupid when you take something they struggle with and turn it upside down to solve the problem in no time. *No one* peels a banana that way."

"I don't know why not, made sense to me," replied Ms. Smart. Ms. Smart does not place great value on respecting accepted behaviors, authority, and tradition. It is an unconscious part of the way she conducts herself. It never occurs to her that she shouldn't question accepted rules. Her spouse, on the other hand, respects them. It rarely occurs to him that he should question them.

He and Ms. Smart have some interesting discussion.

"So you are saying that the way I peel a banana or solve a problem can create hostility, even when people want it peeled or solved?"

"Yes," he said.

"So, if I want to maintain good relationships, I have to be sensitive to whether or not peeling a banana upside down might contradict their values, and not be so abrupt with it?"

"That seems the case to me," he said.

"That wastes so much time!"

"Well," he suggested, "I guess it depends on your values. If you need their cooperation to reach your goals, it may be your best investment of time."

"I hate having to dance around feelings," she protested. "But I think you have something there. I'll just have to decide what I value most and act accordingly."

Conclusion

Values affect the jobs people do and the way they do those jobs. Just go into any organization populated with employees whose only goal is to put in time until retirement. Then go into a medical practice whose employees are committed to taking care of patients and making the organization thrive. You can see, hear, and feel the difference.

It is essential to clarify your values so you can take care of yourself and then take care of your organization. Clarifying values determines the options available to managers who are caught in the middle. The best place to clarify those values *is* in the middle — where powerful, and sometimes opposing, forces pull and push health care, your organization, and your career.

Consider the conflicts and challenges of the middle as your friends, not your enemies. They signal the need to clarify values, and they can be your teachers in the hard work of doing so. In the melting pot of the workplace, a wonderful brew of human interaction can be found. Differing values and dialogue are flavorings in that brew.

CONCLUSION

You don't have to carry the weight of the world

Managers are always caught in the middle. It goes with the position. As managers, we work with contradictory and sometimes mutually exclusive demands. We always have to translate between the boss and employees, and direct our organizations between today's realities and tomorrow's possibilities. Our jobs are to walk into chaos and make things as right as possible. That's why employers hire us. Without those pressures, many of us would not have jobs. With those pressures, many of us feel caught in the middle, in a no-win situation.

Dr. Ed Hampe, our clinical psychologist friend, is fond of saying, "The truth will make you free, but first it will make you miserable." So, in this book the authors have told you some things we believe to be true, knowing full well that some of them may disturb you. At the same time, we have also told you what we believe to be effective ways of dealing with those truths. That combination frees you to do productive work.

The disturbing truth is that health care, your job, and your employer are all changing radically and rapidly. We are not nearing the end of changes; we are closer to the beginning. In addition to the usual demands of management, you may well have the burden of job changes, new employers, new responsibilities, and even the possibility of unemployment. Add the chaos of health care changes, the pressures of family responsibilities, and the sensitivity of personal issues to those demands, and as a manager of a medical practice, you are tired and you may be at risk. It's easy to feel like Atlas — not sure you can hold the world up any longer, yet unable to set it down.

Our message is clear and simple. First, take care of yourself. Then, you can take care of your organization, if it can be taken care of, and if it deserves to be taken care of. The "if" statements are our way of saying that it is not necessary to carry the weight of the world. You *can* lay the burden aside, and sometimes, it may make sense to drop it.

We believe your first obligation is to yourself. If you are happy and productive, your organization will benefit as a by-product.

OhmygoshthisbookdescribesmeIhopeitsnottrue!

The most difficult thing about being caught in the middle may be acknowledging the truth about health care today. Just say, "OK, that's how it is. I'm between the rock and the hard place, between the devil and the deep blue sea," and to quote a manager who mixes metaphors, "up the creek on thin ice."

Taking care of yourself and taking care of your organization is a matter of accepting some truths and then changing some habitual ways of thinking, feeling, and acting.

As managers, we are paid to take care of our organizations. The simple, overriding fact is that we can't do that without first taking care of ourselves.

ABOUT the AUTHORS

CLYDE W. JACKSON is a management and human resources consultant in Louisville, Ky. Mr. Jackson earned a B.S. in Psychology from Ouachita Baptist University in Arkadelphia, Ark., and an M.Div., from the Southern Baptist Theological Seminary in Louisville, Ky., with additional study at the University of Iowa and the University of Louisville. His consulting practice focuses on organizational effectiveness, executive development, client satisfaction, self-managed teams, and problem intervention. His clients include medical services management companies, manufacturers, long-term care facilities, academic institutions, retailers, food service companies, and not-for-profit organizations. Previous writings include three books, business journal articles, and a weekly newspaper column. He is a frequent speaker and seminar leader. He co-authored *From Green Persimmons to Cranky Parrots.*

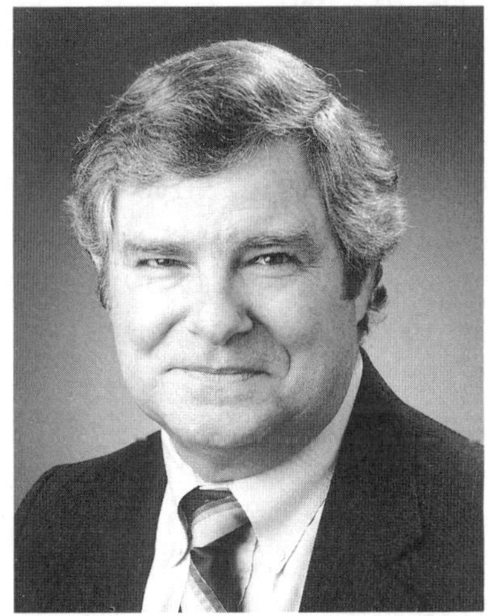

ROBERT SLATON, Ed.D., FACMPE, is the Associate Vice President for Ambulatory Care at the University of Louisville School of Medicine, Louisville, Ky. In that capacity he serves as the director of both the University's teaching clinics, through its Primary Care Center, and the faculty practice group. Dr. Slaton previously served as Administrator for External Affairs at Trover Clinic, a large multi-specialty group practice. He is also a former Commissioner of Health for the Commonwealth of Kentucky. He holds faculty appointments in family and community medicine and psychiatry and behavior sciences, and annually teaches a health policy and practice management course to fourth-year medical students. He also occasionally teaches management courses for both the University's School of Social Work and its School of Business and Public Administration. Dr. Slaton is a frequent speaker on practice management, health care administration, health care reform, managed care, and public health. He earned his degree in Educational Administration at the University of Louisville. Active in MGMA for more than 10 years, he is a Fellow of the American College of Medical Practice Executives. He co-authored the book *From Green Persimmons to Cranky Parrots.*

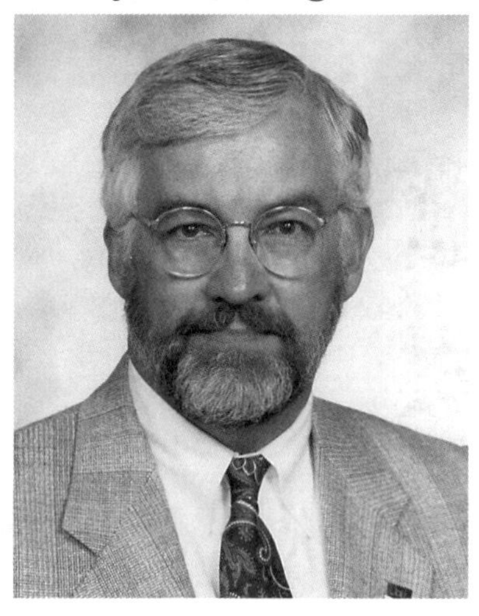

BOB MANNING is a Practice Administrator for Community Medical Associates, a 22-physician group in Louisville, Ky. Previously he was a marketing and software specialist for a custom programming company, and he taught computer courses at the University of Louisville. His earlier career includes positions as a general business consultant for a private consulting firm, and many years work in mangement and marketing positions in the not-for-profit and arts sector. With a degree in English from Bellarmine College, Mr. Manning has wide experience writing and editing technical documentation for computer users, and he is the author of numerous marketing pieces for both print and electronic media. Mr. Manning is a published playwright whose work has been produced both in this country and abroad. He is a member of the Medical Group Management Association (MGMA), and is a Nominee in the American College of Medical Practice Executives (ACMPE). Mr. Manning is a co-author of the book *From Green Persimmons to Cranky Parrots* published by MGMA in 1993.

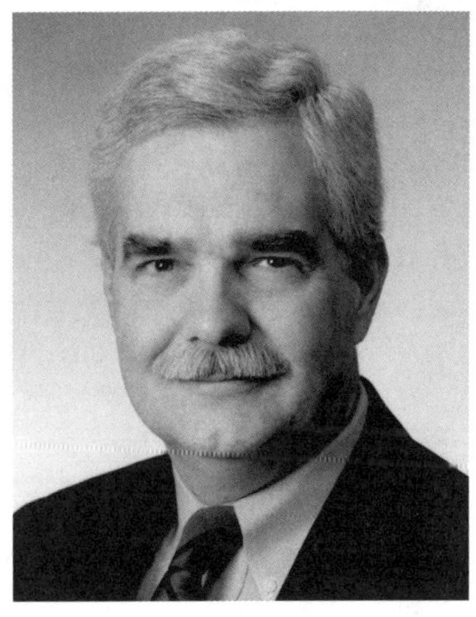

L**YLE SLATON** attended courses at Eastern Kentucky University and is enrolled in a paramedic training program at Commonwealth Ambulance Service, the largest private ambulance service in the State of Kentucky. He is currently employed as an emergency medical technician. Lyle also illustrated *From Green Persimmons to Cranky Parrots*, co-authored by his father Robert Slaton. Lyle's hobbies include art, building military models and studying military history.

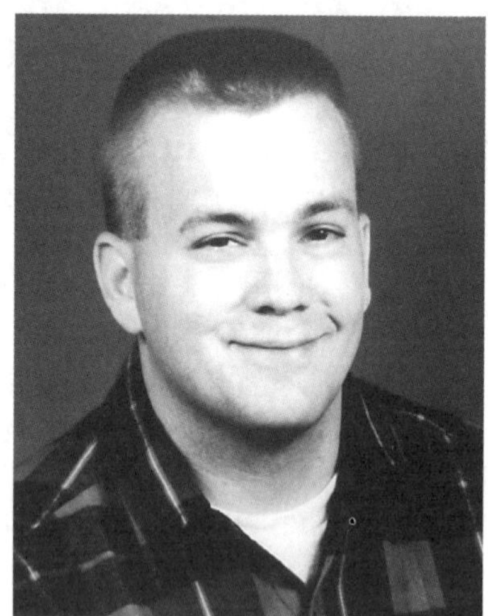